Image-Guided Spine Interventions

Guest Editor

JOHN M. MATHIS, MD, MSc

NEUROIMAGING CLINICS OF NORTH AMERICA

www.neuroimaging.theclinics.com

Consulting Editor

SURESH K. MUKHERJI, MD

May 2010 • Volume 20 • Number 2

SAUNDERS an imprint of ELSEVIER, Inc.

W.B. SAUNDERS COMPANY
A Division of Elsevier Inc.

1600 John F. Kennedy Boulevard ● Suite 1800 ● Philadelphia, Pennsylvania 19103-2899

http://www.theclinics.com

NEUROIMAGING CLINICS OF NORTH AMERICA Volume 20, Number 2
May 2010 ISSN 1052-5149, ISBN 13: 978-1-4377-2271-0

Editor: Joanne Husovski
Developmental Editor: Theresa Collier

Neuroimaging Clinics of North America (ISSN 1052-5149) is published quarterly by Elsevier Inc., 360 Park Avenue South, New York, NY 10010-1710. Months of issue are February, May, August, and November. Business and editorial offices: 1600 John F. Kennedy Blvd., Suite 1800, Philadelphia, PA 19103-2899. Business and editorial offices: 6277 Sea Harbor Drive, Orlando, FL 32887-4800. Periodicals postage paid at New York, NY, and additional mailing offices. Subscription prices are USD 293 per year for US individuals, USD 415 per year for US institutions, USD 150 per year for US students and residents, USD 339 per year for Canadian individuals, USD 520 per year for Canadian institutions, USD 431 per year for international individuals, USD 520 per year for international institutions and USD 215 per year for Canadian and foreign students and residents. To receive student/resident rate, orders must be accompanied by name of affiliated institution, date of term, and the *signature* of program/residency coordinator on institution letterhead. Orders will be billed at individual rate until proof of status is received. Foreign air speed delivery is included in all *Clinics* subscription prices. All prices are subject to change without notice. POSTMASTER: Send address changes to *Neuroimaging Clinics of North America*, Elsevier Health Sciences Division, Subscription Customer Service, 3251 Riverport Lane, Maryland Heights, MO 63043. Telephone: 1-800-654-2452 (U.S. and Canada); 314-447-8871 (outside U.S. and Canada). Fax: 314-447-8029. E-mail: journalscustomerservice-usa@elsevier.com (for print support); journalsonlinesupport-usa@elsevier.com (for online support).

Reprints. For copies of 100 or more of articles in this publication, please contact the Commercial Reprints Department, Elsevier Inc., 360 Park Avenue South, New York, NY 10010-1710. Tel.: 212-633-3812; Fax: 212-462-1935; E-mail: reprints@elsevier.com.

Neuroimaging Clinics of North America is covered by *Excerpta Medical/EMBASE,* the RSNA Index of Imaging Literature, *MEDLINE/PubMed (Index Medicus),* MEDLINE/MEDLARS, SciSearch, Research Alert, and Neuroscience Citation Index.

Printed and bound in the United Kingdom
Transferred to Digital Print 2011

GOAL STATEMENT

The goal of *Neuroimaging Clinics of North America* is to keep practicing radiologists and radiology residents up to date with current clinical practice in radiology by providing timely articles reviewing the state of the art in patient care.

ACCREDITATION

The *Neuroimaging Clinics of North America* is planned and implemented in accordance with the Essential Areas and Policies of the Accreditation Council for Continuing Medical Education (ACCME) through the joint sponsorship of the University of Virginia School of Medicine and Elsevier. The University of Virginia School of Medicine is accredited by the ACCME to provide continuing medical education for physicians.

The University of Virginia School of Medicine designates this educational activity for a maximum of 15 *AMA PRA Category 1 Credits*™ for each issue, 60 credits per year. Physicians should only claim credit commensurate with the extent of their participation in the activity.

The American Medical Association has determined that physicians not licensed in the US who participate in this CME activity are eligible for a maximum of 15 *AMA PRA Category 1 Credits*™ for each issue, 60 credits per year.

Credit can be earned by reading the text material, taking the CME examination online at http://www.theclinics.com/home/cme, and completing the evaluation. After taking the test, you will be required to review any and all incorrect answers. Following completion of the test and evaluation, your credit will be awarded and you may print your certificate.

FACULTY DISCLOSURE/CONFLICT OF INTEREST

The University of Virginia School of Medicine, as an ACCME accredited provider, endorses and strives to comply with the Accreditation Council for Continuing Medical Education (ACCME) Standards of Commercial Support, Commonwealth of Virginia statutes, University of Virginia policies and procedures, and associated federal and private regulations and guidelines on the need for disclosure and monitoring of proprietary and financial interests that may affect the scientific integrity and balance of content delivered in continuing medical education activities under our auspices.

The University of Virginia School of Medicine requires that all CME activities accredited through this institution be developed independently and be scientifically rigorous, balanced and objective in the presentation/discussion of its content, theories and practices.

All authors/editors participating in an accredited CME activity are expected to disclose to the readers relevant financial relationships with commercial entities occurring within the past 12 months (such as grants or research support, employee, consultant, stock holder, member of speakers bureau, etc.). The University of Virginia School of Medicine will employ appropriate mechanisms to resolve potential conflicts of interest to maintain the standards of fair and balanced education to the reader. Questions about specific strategies can be directed to the Office of Continuing Medical Education, University of Virginia School of Medicine, Charlottesville, Virginia.

The faculty and staff of the University of Virginia Office of Continuing Medical Education have no financial affiliations to disclose.

The authors/editors listed below have identified no professional/financial affiliations for themselves or their spouse/partner:
Omer Abdulrehman Awan, MD; Giuseppe Bonaldi, MD; Charles H. Cho, MD, MBA; Celene Hadley, MD; Joanne Husovski (Acquisitions Editor); Lubda M. Shah, MD (Test Author); and Gregg H. Zoarski, MD.

The authors listed below have identified the following professional/financial affiliations for themselves or their spouse/partner:
Bassem A. Georgy, MD is an industry funded research/investigator and consultant, and serves on the Speakers' Bureau for Arthrocare and DePuy Spine; is a patent holder for DePuy Spine; and owns stock for Osseon LLC, Spine Aligns, and Dfine.
Stanley Golovac, MD is a consultant and serves on the Speakers Bureau for Stryker Corporation, and is a consultant, serves on the Speakers Bureau, and serves on the Advisory Committee/Board for St. Jude Medical.
John M. Mathis, MD, MSc (Guest Editor) serves on the Advisory Committee/Board for Orthovita and Bromimetics, and is employed by the FDA.
Suresh K. Mukherji, MD (Consulting Editor) is a consultant for Philips.
Orlando Ortiz, MD, MBA is a consultant for SpineWave, Inc., and is on the Speakers' Bureau for Medtronic Spine.

Disclosure of Discussion of Non-FDA Approved Uses for Pharmaceutical Products and/or Medical Devices.
The University of Virginia School of Medicine, as an ACCME provider, requires that all faculty presenters identify and disclose any off-label uses for pharmaceutical and medical device products. The University of Virginia School of Medicine recommends that each physician fully review all the available data on new products or procedures prior to clinical use.

TO ENROLL

To enroll in the Neuroimaging Clinics of North America Continuing Medical Education program, call customer service at 1-800-654-2452 or sign up online at *http://www.theclinics.com/home/cme*. The CME program is available to subscribers for an additional annual fee of USD 175.

Neuroimaging Clinics of North America

THE CLINICS ARE NOW AVAILABLE ONLINE!

Access your subscription at:
www.theclinics.com

Contributors

CONSULTING EDITOR

SURESH K. MUKHERJI, MD
Professor and Chief of Neuroradiology
and Head and Neck Radiology; Professor
of Radiology, Otolaryngology Head and Neck
Surgery and Radiation Oncology, University
of Michigan Health System, Ann Arbor,
Michigan

GUEST EDITOR

JOHN M. MATHIS, MD, MSc
Past President, American Society of Spine
Radiology; Medical Director, Centers for
Advanced Imaging, Roanoke, Virginia

AUTHORS

OMER ABDULREHMAN AWAN, MD
Radiology Resident, University of Maryland
Medical Center, Baltimore, Maryland

GIUSEPPE BONALDI, MD
Director, Department of Neuroradiology, Riuniti
Hospital, Bergamo, Italy

CHARLES H. CHO, MD, MBA
Department of Radiology, Brigham and
Women's Hospital, Harvard Medical School,
Boston, Massachusetts

BASSEM A. GEORGY, MD
North County Radiology, Escondido,
California; Assistant Professor, Department
of Radiology, University of California, San
Diego, California

STANLEY GOLOVAC, MD
Co-director of Space Coast Pain Institute,
Consultant for Stryker Corporation and for
Spinal Restoration, St. Jude Medical Neuro
Division, Merritt Island, Florida

CELENE HADLEY, MD
Neuroradiology Fellow, University of Maryland
Medical Center, Baltimore, Maryland

JOHN M. MATHIS, MD, MSc
Past President, American Society of Spine
Radiology; Medical Director, Centers for
Advanced Imaging, Roanoke, Virginia

ORLANDO ORTIZ, MD, MBA, FACR
Chairman, Department of Radiology,
Winthrop-University Hospital, Mineola,
New York; Professor of Clinical Radiology,
School of Medicine, Stony Brook University,
Stony Brook, New York

GREGG H. ZOARSKI, MD
Associate Professor of Diagnostic Radiology
and Nuclear Medicine; Director,
Neuroradiology, Division of Neurosciences,
University of Maryland Medical Center,
Baltimore, Maryland

Contents

> Vertebral augmentation techniques use image guidance for the percutaneous place-
> ment of spinal implants that stabilize a painful osteoporotic or pathologic vertebral
> compression fracture. The initial implant, acrylic bone cement, was injected through
> a bone needle into the vertebral body, a procedure referred to as vertebroplasty.
> A modification of this procedure, kyphoplasty, entails the temporary use of an inflat-
> able balloon tamp before cement injection. Other techniques and the equipment
> required to perform these vertebral augmentation procedures have evolved signifi-
> cantly during the past two decades. It is now possible to perform vertebral body re-
> construction in patients with painful fractures of compromised vertebrae with
> excellent outcomes in terms of sustainable pain relief and marked reduction in pa-
> tient morbidity.

> Percutaneous vertebral augmentation is a successful means of relieving pain and re-
> ducing disability after vertebral compression fracture; however, the exact mecha-
> nism by which vertebral augmentation eliminates pain remains unproven. Most
> likely, pain relief is because of stabilization of microfractures. The biomechanical ef-
> fects of vertebral fracture and subsequent vertebral augmentation therapy, however,
> are topics for continued investigation. Altered biomechanical stresses after treat-
> ment may affect the risk of adjacent fracture in an osteoporotic patient; that risk
> may be different after vertebral augmentation with cavity creation (balloon assisted
> vertebroplasty or kyphoplasty) when compared with vertebral augmentation without
> cavity creation (vertebroplasty). Polymethyl methacrylate cement used in these pro-
> cedures may have an important effect on the load transfer and disk mechanics, and
> therefore, the variables of cement volume, formulation, and distribution should also
> be evaluated. Finally, the question of whether prophylactic treatment of adjacent in-
> tact levels is indicated must be considered.

> The purpose of this article is to review the current state of the art of using vertebral
> augmentation techniques for treating symptomatic spinal fractures that are associ-
> ated with malignant lesions and to present potential future trends in treatments for
> this patient population. Epidemiology and biomechanical ramifications of these
> lesions are summarized, and treatment regimes, clinical outcomes, complications,
> and technical issues associated with treatments are presented. Potential future
> trends and new technologies for performing vertebral body augmentation in patients
> with metastatic spinal lesions are also discussed in this article.

Pain from sacral insufficiency fractures or metastatic tumor to the sacrum, refractory to radiation and/or chemotherapy, can be extremely debilitating to affected patients. Conservative medical therapy with rest, limited ambulation, and pain medication has been the mainstay of treatment. Open surgical fixation is reserved for severe fracture that does not heal with rest. A minimally invasive treatment, sacroplasty, is gaining popularity and uses image-guided, percutaneous injection of surgical cement into the fracture. This article reviews the incidence, causes, diagnosis, presentation, and treatment options for sacral fractures, and describes detailed technical steps of the sacroplasty procedure.

Synovial cysts have long been known to create radicular pain in the spine, with the clinical effect mimicking a disk herniation. These cysts have traditionally been treated with open surgical therapy. Now a minimally invasive, image-guided approach to treatment is available to relieve this problem, using a simple percutaneous needle stick and injection. This article describes the technical aspects and precautions needed for this intervention.

Epidural steroid injections have been used for decades as part of a rehabilitation program to relieve back or neck pain and the associated radicular nerve component that often accompanies these problems. These injections are minimally invasive and offer many patients substantial relief without the need for more invasive procedures. Although effective and generally simple, they must be performed accurately and properly for maximum benefit and complication avoidance. This article discusses the various technical aspects of the procedure that must be observed by the operator to accomplish these ends.

Pain that develops in the cervical, thoracic, lumbar, and sacral spine is typically initiated from a clinical condition called spondylosis. Radiofrequency ablation is a key element in the treatment protocol of patients with spondylosis of the cervical, thoracic, lumbar, and sacroiliac joint pain. A diagnosis can be made by blocking the median branch nerve that innervates each joint. Once this has been confirmed, an ablation procedure can be performed to increase the duration of pain relief desired by the patient with chronic pain originating from spondylosis. Radiofrequency neurolysis is a common technique used in the treatment of chronic pain, particularly facet (zygapophyseal joint) arthralgia. The technique involves an insulated needlelike cannula; x-rays passing through the patient show the projected relative radioopaque bony landmarks and the metallic cannula.

As image-guided (nonvascular) spine interventions have become progressively more common in the interventional radiologic community, there is a growing need for physician expertise regarding the materials and pharmaceuticals that are used for these procedures. This article is intended to provide information to address these needs.

Percutaneous lumbar discectomy is a proven alternative to the more invasive open discectomy used to treat patients who experience discogenic pain. Estimated to cost the United States health care system more than $20 billion a year, discogenic leg pain represents the primary cause of health care expenditure. Taken together, back pain and discogenic leg pain result in more days lost than any other combined illnesses and injuries. Annular breakdown and tears are common discogenic sources that produce pain, and are usually treated with microdiscectomy by orthopedic surgeons and neurosurgeons. Open discectomy has been considered to be the gold standard for relieving pressure on nerve roots. By decompressing the nerve root from the disc, neurologic function is usually restored and pain is relieved. Recurrent disc herniations may and typically do occur because of the annular violation that results from the surgical procedure.

Fusion techniques are considered the gold standard for treatment of lumbar spinal instability, although there are many shortcomings and disadvantages. In the past two decades the concept of dynamic stabilization has been introduced in clinical practice. A more thorough knowledge of the spinal biomechanics has led to the ability to modify the loads within the spinal unit. Many different devices based on this concept were designed. Almost all these devices are percutaneous or minimally invasive. Thus, not only surgeons but also interventional radiologists can play a major role in the treatment of the degenerated spine.

Spinal cord stimulation has been used successfully for more than 40 years. The application of an electrical impulse field on to the spinal cord is used with a battery generator source and a variety of either cylindrical or paddle/plate leads. Energy is delivered from either a conventional internal programmable generator or a rechargeable style battery. Many clinical conditions such as complex regional pain syndrome, failed back spinal syndrome, and extremity neuropathic pain involving the trunk and limbs are approved for its use. This device allows patients to live a successful life without pain.

Preface

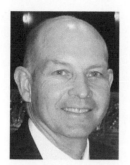

John M. Mathis, MD, MSc
Guest Editor

The neurologic system is generally divided into the brain and spinal cord, along with the associated supporting or protective structures (the skull and spinal column). In medical literature, more is written about the brain and, indeed, in referral centers more diagnostic and therapeutic time is spent with this part of the neurologic system than any other. However, a greater portion of the public requires therapy for spine because of pain and disability. Fortunately, the problems that most patients experience are not life threatening; nevertheless, they are commonly disabling and life altering.

Both diagnostic imaging and minimally invasive image-guided therapy for spine-related problems have improved and evolved over the course of the last two decades. Today, we not only have the ability to identify a specific source of pain, we have focused treatments that can be applied to address or repair problems that exist. The therapeutic evolution was carried forward by the pioneering work of our diagnostic colleagues who provided us with the means of visualizing the problems that plague our patients. Following this imaging awareness has been the development of pharmaceuticals, materials, and devices that can be used to provide minimally invasive (often with a simple percutaneous needle placement) therapy for numerous conditions. These conditions include intervertebral disc disease, spinal stenosis, facet degenerative disease, synovial cyst formation, and fractures or malignant destruction of vertebral bodies and sacrum. Diagnosis is aided by selective image-guided biopsy.

This edition of the *Neuroimaging Clinics* focuses on these minimally invasive, image-guided therapies. It includes guidelines for patient assessment and selection, choices of pharmaceuticals and materials commonly used, and advice from noted experts about complication avoidance. Common procedures such as biopsy, epidural steroid injection, and vertebroplasty (or balloon-assisted vertebroplasty) are discussed. Newer procedures, such as sacroplasty, synovial cyst rupture, spinal cord stimulators, neurolysis, percutaneous discectomy, and minimally invasive treatment of spinal stenosis, are introduced.

Physicians providing minimally invasive spine therapies and spine pain management will obtain valuable information from this resource. Additionally, diagnostic physicians will benefit by knowing the available therapies that can be recommended to patients who have diseases that can be treated with the minimally invasive procedures discussed in this issue.

John M. Mathis, MD, MSc
Center for Advanced Imaging
Roanoke, VA 24014, USA

E-mail address:
jmathis@rev.net

Neuroimag Clin N Am 20 (2010) xi
doi:10.1016/j.nic.2010.02.011

Preface

Image-Guided Spine Interventions

Vertebral Body Reconstruction: Techniques and Tools

Orlando Ortiz, MD, MBA[a,b], John M. Mathis, MD, MSc[c,*]

KEYWORDS

- Vertebroplasty • Kyphoplasty
- Osteoporotic vertebral compression fractures

Vertebroplasty and kyphoplasty are both standard-of-care procedures for the treatment of painful osteoporotic and pathologic vertebral compression fractures of the spinal axis.[1] This article reviews the evolution of these treatments in the context of vertebral body reconstruction. Technical developments and improvements in vertebral augmentation are also discussed.

Several decades have passed since the first case of vertebroplasty was performed.[2] Although this case entailed a transoral approach and the target lesion was a painful C2 aggressive hemangioma, a fundamental principle of the vertebroplasty procedure was used, which is pain relief through vertebral body stabilization as a consequence of image-guided bone needle placement and the subsequent injection of acrylic bone cement (polymethylmethacrylate).[3] As shown in numerous prospective and retrospective studies, vertebroplasty is a safe and effective procedure for treating painful osteoporotic or pathologic fractures of the spinal axis.[4–6] Nearly one decade after percutaneous vertebroplasty (PV) was in use, balloon-assisted vertebroplasty, or kyphoplasty, was developed with the goal of osteoporotic vertebral compression fracture reduction and kyphosis correction.[7,8] Like vertebroplasty, kyphoplasty entails image-guided percutaneous bone needle

placement. A bone needle is placed through either a transpedicular or a parapedicular route from either a bilateral or a unilateral approach. In kyphoplasty, before cement injection, a working cavity is created in the target vertebra by temporarily inflating and then removing a balloon tamp.[9] In acute and early subacute fractures, the balloon tamp Is capable of elevating the depressed vertebral endplate.[10–13] A review of the published literature shows that kyphoplasty is an effective treatment for painful osteoporotic and pathologic vertebral compression fractures.[6,14] In the more than two decades of the vertebroplasty procedure, thousands of patients have been successfully treated as evidenced by a significant relief of their back pain symptoms, reduction of analgesic use, and return to normal activities of daily living. Furthermore, for those patients who were initially so debilitated that they required hospitalization for pain management, these procedures have resulted in a marked reduction in hospital length of stay, with quick progression to rehabilitation therapy.

(Editor's Note: There is considerable controversy about whether any real advantage of kyphoplasty over percutaneous vertebroplasty exists. Vertebroplasty is much less expensive

Disclosures: Speakers Bureau, Medtronic Spine (Memphis TN); Consultant, SpineWave Inc (Shelton, CT) (OO); Consultant, Food and Drug Administration, Division of Orthopedics and Rehabilitation Medicine (injectable biomaterials); Consultant, Orthovita Inc, Malvern, PA; Orthopedic Advisory Board, Biomimetic Therapeutics; Advisory Board/Consultant, Crosstrees Medical Inc; Advisory Board, Graduate School of Biomedical Engineering (Wake Forest University/ Virginia Tech University) (JM).
a Department of Radiology, Winthrop-University Hospital, 259 First Street, Mineola, NY 11501, USA
b Stony Brook University School of Medicine, Stony Brook, NY, USA
c Center for Advanced Imaging, Roanoke, VA 24014, USA
* Corresponding author.
E-mail address: jmathis@rev.net

Neuroimag Clin N Am 20 (2010) 145–158
doi:10.1016/j.nic.2010.02.001

neuroimaging.theclinics.com

and therefore has a decided advantage if no benefit of kyphoplasty otherwise exists. A position paper by multiple societies in Radiology and Neurosurgery concludes "There is no proved advantage of kyphoplasty relative to vertebroplasty with regard to pain relief, vertebral height restoration, or complications." J Vasc Interv Radiol 2007;18:325–30.)

Vertebroplasty and kyphoplasty are the vertebral augmentation procedures that are used to treat vertebral bodies that are compromised by either an osteoporotic collapse or a neoplastic infiltration. Vertebral augmentation is the stabilization of a damaged vertebra with the placement of an implant (acrylic bone cement as the first approved agent) within the anterior column of the vertebral body. In the specific case of sacroplasty, acrylic bone cement is injected into the sacral ala to augment sacral lesions, such as sacral insufficiency fractures. Kyphoplasty reflected a change not only in the equipment required to perform vertebral augmentation but also in the treatment goal of the procedure, the vertebral compression fracture reduction through vertebral body reconstruction. Vertebral body reconstruction attempts to restore the morphologic and structural integrity of the vertebral body. The damaged vertebra is remodeled before the placement of an implant. The objective of this procedure is to maximally restore the biomechanical properties of the treated vertebra. A working cavity is created within the vertebral body using the balloon tamp and, at times, a curette. Attempts are made to repair and restore the alignment of the vertebral endplates.

Not all vertebral compression fractures are the same. These fractures occur at different locations of the spinal axis, such as the midthoracic spine (T5–T8), the thoracolumbar junction (T10–L2), or the sacrum. These fractures are the result of varying severities of osteoporosis, osteonecrosis, or neoplastic infiltration, all of which compromise the load-bearing trabecular and cortical matrix of the vertebral body. The morphologic and structural alterations that are present can likewise be variable. Furthermore, osteoporotic fractures can be acute, subacute, or chronic. Chronic fractures may have healed, albeit in a deformed state, and may not be an actual source of pain. Similarly, host factors (comorbidities, patient activity level before sustaining the fracture, preexisting spine conditions) in patients with vertebral compression fractures are obviously variable. Given these observations, it is not surprising that several instruments and implants have been developed to treat this less than homogeneous group of patients.

Advances in vertebral body reconstruction techniques can be categorized into 6 major types:

1. Bone access needles
2. Cavity creation devices
3. Coaxial cement conduits
4. Cement delivery systems
5. Implants
6. Pathologic fracture treatment.

These advancements have occurred in an attempt to improve the efficiency, effectiveness, and safety of the vertebral augmentation procedure. The objective of vertebral augmentation, after all, is to place the implant within the vertebral body, avoiding, for example, implant migration such as cement extravasation and providing optimal anterior column stabilization.

BONE ACCESS

Developments in percutaneous bone needle access have focused primarily on curved needles (Fig. 1). These needles have either a fixed curve or an adjustable curve to control directionality. The advantage of curved needle technology is the ability to use only a unilateral approach via a single skin puncture.[15] A second potential advantage of curved needle technology is the selective placement of the needle tip into predetermined target areas of the damaged vertebra, with delivery of the implant to the targets. Because they are deployed through a straight guide cannula or have adjustable curves, these curved needles have somewhat flexible tips that do not always precisely navigate through the vertebral body. Clogging of the needle lumen with hardening cement may occur, requiring removal of the needle. The theoretical potential for breakage of the needle tip or cementing of the needle into the vertebra must be avoided.

CAVITY CREATION

Several devices that can create a working cavity for subsequent implant deposition have been developed for clinical use. The first of these devices, a bone curette, was developed for the kyphoplasty procedure (Fig. 2). This curette possesses an adjustable wedge or mushroom-shaped tip that can be angled up to 90°, in 30° increments, relative to the shaft of the device. The curette, however, must be used with an 8-gauge guide cannula. Another cavity-creation device has a tip that can be variably adjusted to 90° and can be placed through a 10-gauge guide cannula (OpitMed, Ettlingen, Germany). Both of these devices have a built-in

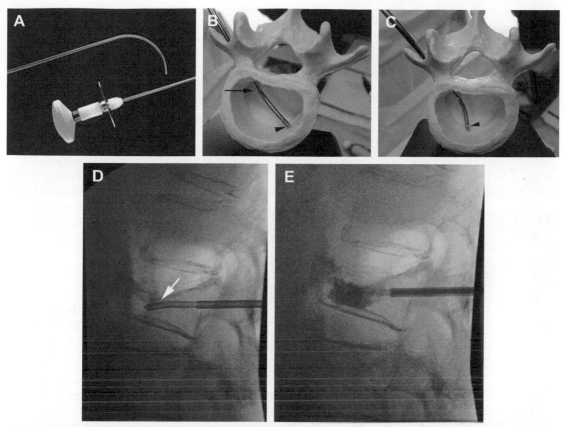

Fig. 1. Bone needles. (*A*) Curved nitinol stylet of a curved needle (*Courtesy of* Cook Medical, Inc, Bloomington, IN; with permission). (*B, C*) A curved needle (*arrows*) can be manipulated to multiple areas within a vertebral body through a transpedicular approach as shown in the sawbones model (Cardinal Health, Inc, Dublin, OH). (*D, E*) Lateral radiographs of the spine before and during cement injection in a vertebroplasty procedure with a curved needle (*arrow in D*) placed into a wedge compression deformity of a lower thoracic vertebra (Osseon Therapeutics, Inc, Santa Rosa, CA).

fail-safe mechanism that allows the sculpting tip to remain attached in a neutral position, thus allowing device extraction, when the device tip breaks within the sclerotic bone.

Another cavity-creation device uses an adjustable flexible tip with variable angulation; this device must be deployed through a guiding cannula (see **Fig. 2**). Other fixed-tip systems are available for use as well; the smallest of these can be deployed through a 10.5-gauge–sized cannula (see **Fig. 2**). A goal for cavity creation is to facilitate controlled implant delivery. The clear advantage of this maneuver is that it minimizes or prevents extravertebral migration of the implant, in particular cement extravasation with its adverse consequences. Cavity creation is a form of vertebral body remodeling, but in and of itself does not result in correction of vertebral endplate deformities or restoration of vertebral body height loss.

(Editor's note: There are now reports that cavity creation can actually weaken the bone by removing its residual bone elements compressed during the process of compression fracture. Constructs such as those created with Kyphon may be weaker, and therefore subsequently loose height gained compared to Vertebroplasty; eg, Kim MJ, Lindsey DP, Hannibal M, et al. Vertebroplasty versus kyphoplasty: biomedical behavior under repetitive loading conditions. Spine 2006;31:2079–84).

COAXIAL CEMENT CONDUITS

Coaxial cement conduits were first used with the kyphoplasty procedure (**Fig. 3**). These bone-filler devices facilitate controlled implant delivery. In the case of the acrylic bone cement,

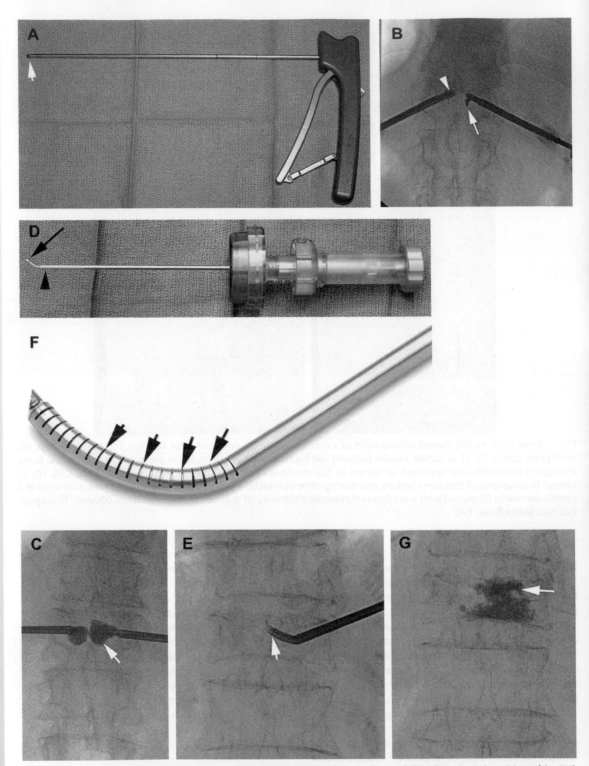

Fig. 2. Bone curettes. (*A*) A bone curette with adjustable wedge tip (*arrow*) (Medtronic Spine, Memphis, TN). (*B, C*) Frontal radiographs of the spine showing use of curette (*arrow in B*) to facilitate balloon tamp inflation (*arrow in C*) in a chronic fracture; note lack of balloon inflation (*arrowhead in B*) before the use of the curette. (*D*) A fixed curette (*arrowhead*) that is inserted coaxially through a guiding cannula (*arrowhead*) (ArthroCare Spine, Austin, TX). (*E, F, G*) Frontal radiograph of spine showing use of an adjustable curette (*arrow in E*) with close-up photograph of the curette tip (*F*) and facilitated cement injection during vertebroplasty (*G*) (DFine Corp, San Jose, CA).

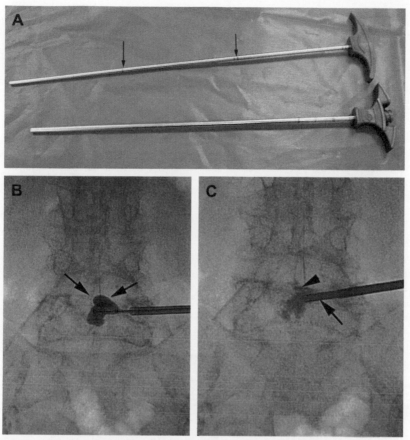

Fig. 3. Coaxial cement cannulas. (A) A bone-filler device that holds 1.5 mL of acrylic bone cement; the stylet has 0.5 mL markings (arrows) (Medtronic Spine, Memphis, TN). (B) Frontal radiograph of the spine during balloon tamp inflation showing large endplate defect (arrows). (C) Frontal radiograph of the spine during injection with very thick cement through the bone-filler device (arrow) showing closure of the endplate defect (arrowhead).

they prevent obstruction or occlusion of the primary needle cannula with hardened cement. Access to the vertebral body is maintained, and the operator is not pressured to administer acrylic bone cement in a shorter period of time. Alternatively, the operator can use more viscous cement in situations such as closure of endplate defects that require the use of thicker cement. Thirteen-gauge–sized coaxial cement conduits have been developed for use in the vertebro-plasty procedure using smaller gauge needle systems, such as a 10.5-gauge cannula (Fig. 4). Stylets or plungers, rather than syringes or hydraulic cement delivery systems, can be used to deliver the thicker cement when neces-sary. The cement can be delivered in small 0.2 to 0.3 mL aliquots, using an inject-and-step-back method to significantly reduce the operator radiation exposure during cement injection while at the same time avoiding cement leakage.[16] Use of coaxial cement conduits is a viable,

efficient, and safe alternative for the injection of acrylic bone cement.

CEMENT DELIVERY SYSTEMS

Several types of advancements have taken place with respect to cement delivery systems. The first of these relates to prepackaging of specific dose packs of cement, with premeasured volumes of liquid monomer and polymer powder (Fig. 5). The goal of this change is to improve the consis-tency of the final cement mixture in terms of radio-pacity, viscosity, and working time. Moreover, these ingredients are now mixed in closed systems, often with automated battery-operated mixers to minimize exposure to agents and to improve the likelihood of a consistent cement mix (Fig. 6). A hydraulic system is used with more viscous cement to facilitate controlled cement delivery (Fig. 7). A more recent modifica-tion uses not only a hydraulic system to push the

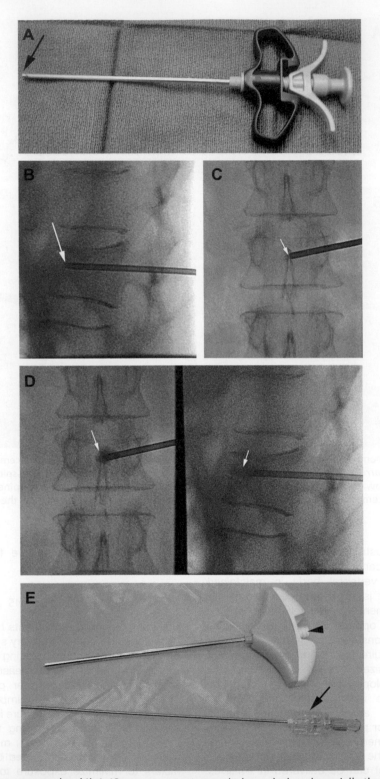

Fig. 4. Coaxial cement cannulas. (*A*) A 13-gauge cement cannula (*arrow*) placed coaxially through a 10.5-gauge bone needle (Stryker Spine, Allendale, NJ). (*B*) Lateral radiograph of the spine during insertion of this cannula (*arrow*). (*C*) Frontal radiograph of the spine during insertion of this cannula (*arrow*). (*D*) Frontal and lateral radiographs of the spine during initial cement injection (*arrows*). (*E*) Cement conduit (*arrow*) that fits into the bone needle cannula (*arrowhead*) (Cardinal Health, Inc, Dublin, OH).

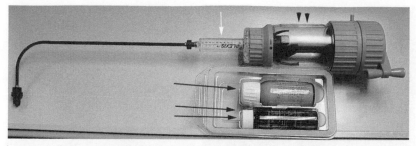

Fig. 5. A closed cement mixing (*arrowheads*) and delivery system (*white arrow*) along with the premeasured amounts of preopacified polymer powder (*arrow*) and liquid monomer (*double arrows*) (Advanced Biomaterials Systems, Chatham, NJ).

thicker cement but also a special radiofrequency pulse to increase viscosity at the time of injection and thereby prolonging the working time of the cement mixture (**Fig. 8**). The use of thicker cement may be useful in situations, such as lytic metastases or large endplate defects, in which the risk of cement extravasation is high.[17] A second advantage is that the hydraulic cement delivery systems allow the operator to stand further away from the fluoroscopy field, thereby reducing

operator radiation exposure. The major disadvantage of all of these systems compared with a simple bowl and palette is their higher cost.

BONE IMPLANTS

Implants that can be used for vertebral body reconstruction include nonbiologic and biologic agents.[18,19] By far, the greatest numbers of vertebral augmentation procedures have been

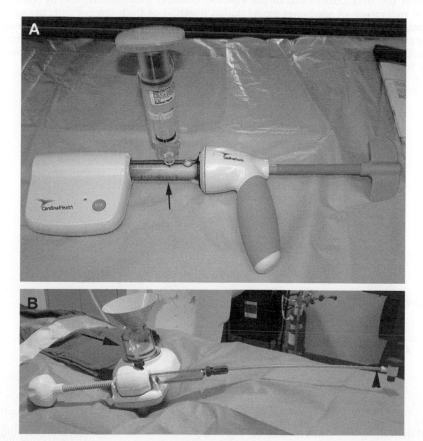

Fig. 6. Automated cement mixing and delivery systems. (*A*) Cement within delivery chamber (*arrow*) (Cardinal Health, Inc, Dublin, OH). (*B*) Another cement delivery system showing the mixing chamber (*arrow*) and the injection tubing (*arrowhead*) (Stryker Spine, Allendale, NJ).

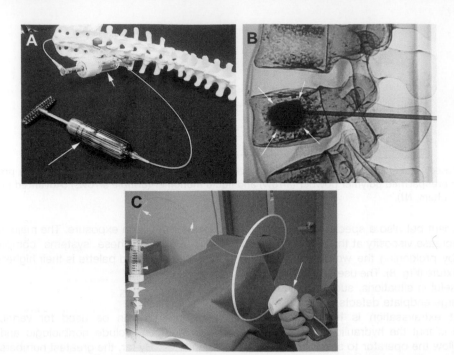

Fig. 7. Hydraulic cement delivery systems. (*A*) A cement delivery system showing the hydraulic chamber (*large arrow*) that forces the thick cement out of the injection chamber (*small arrow*) (DePuy Spine, Inc, Raynham, MA). (*B*) Lateral radiograph of sawbones model during injection of thick cement with the same system as in (*A*) showing controlled cement deposition (*arrows*). (*C*) Another hydraulic system in which the hydraulic pressure is generated by pulling the trigger on the injection gun (*large arrow*) and transmitted via the extra long injection tubing (*small arrows*) to the cement chamber (*arrowhead*) for subsequent extrusion of cement into the bone needle (Medtronic Spine, Memphis, TN).

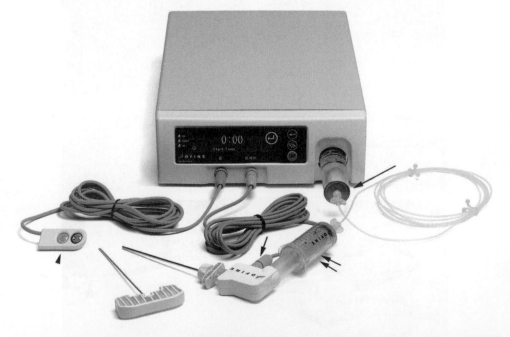

Fig. 8. Cement delivery system that uses a radiofrequency pulse delivered at the injection housing (*small arrow*) to facilitate increased cement viscosity. A hydraulic system (*large arrow*) that pushes the cement in the injection chamber (*double arrows*). The system can be controlled with a plug in the remote device (*arrowhead*) that allows the operator to stand far away from the fluoroscopy field (Dfine Corp, San Jose, CA).

performed with acrylic bone cement. All polymethylmethacrylate cements are now preopacified with barium sulfate for optimal visualization during fluoroscopic monitoring and cement injection. Several biomechanical studies have shown that acrylic bone cement can successfully reinforce a fractured vertebral body and provide strength against axial loading forces. Nevertheless, concerns have been raised about adjacent level fractures in patients recently treated with vertebral augmentation.[20–25] Although this is a somewhat controversial topic in which multiple confounders, including the natural history of osteoporotic vertebral collapse itself, are present, a search for other implants has ensued.

An agent that was recently approved by Food and Drug Administration, Cortoss (Orthovita, Inc, Malvern, PA, USA), consists of a nonresorbable agent that is composed of cross-linked resins and a bioactive glass ceramic, combeite. This agent is radiopaque and is mixed on demand; hence it possesses a very long working time (Fig. 9). Cortoss is osteoconductive, generally requires a smaller injected volume of augmentation material, and preliminary experience suggests that its use may result in a lower adjacent level vertebral fracture rate. The disadvantage of the agent is its cost (recently reduced).

A synthetic hydroxyapatite is also commercially available. This calcium phosphate–based biomaterial is osteoconductive and has increased radiopacity. Two implants are commercially available for the purpose of vertebral body reconstruction. One of these implants consists of polyetheretherketone wafers (Fig. 10). A unilateral extrapedicular approach is required to sequentially stack these wafers using a surgical gun. A small volume of acrylic bone cement is then injected around the wafer stack. In clinical use, this technique demonstrates height restoration and correction of vertebral endplate defects that is maintained at the follow-up. The technique does, however, require the use of a large osteointroducer and access port to deploy the wafers.

Another implant that can be used for vertebral body reconstruction is morcelized bone allograft (Fig. 11). Again, an extrapedicular approach is required to create a large working cavity within the vertebral body using a bone shaver.[26] An acrylic sac is then inserted into the working cavity, and prefilled bone tubes are used to fill the sac with autologous bone graft. Height restoration is achieved through the principle of granular physics. The initial version of the bone cannula was large, but a downsized version is now commercially available. The disadvantage of this system is that the patient is often markedly osteoporotic and may require treatment with an osteogenic medication, with its additional cost and possible side effects.

PATHOLOGIC FRACTURE TREATMENT

Painful pathologic vertebral compression fractures can also be treated with vertebral augmentation techniques. The neoplastic lesions often consist of myeloma or other lytic metastases (Fig. 12). Patients with severe debilitating pain and without spinal cord compromise at the level of the affected vertebra are the potential candidates for these palliative procedures. The procedure may consist of vertebroplasty or kyphoplasty alone or may be preceded by tumor debulking with radiofrequency ablation, plasma-mediated frequency ablation, or cryoablation.[17] The advantage of these procedures over conventional radiation treatment is that they provide immediate pain relief. Furthermore, these procedures can stabilize the pathologically weakened vertebral body, preventing further collapse and potentially preventing spinal canal compromise. A disadvantage of these techniques is that they do not completely eradicate tumor at the treated level; they only treat one specific level, and they carry the risk of spinal canal compromise caused by tumor displacement or cement extravasation.

PAIN RELIEF: REAL VERSUS SHAM CONTROVERSY

With more than 1000 peer-reviewed publications about PV or balloon-assisted vertebroplasty (kyphoplasty) and with hundreds of thousand cases performed, the efficacy of these procedures in terms of pain relief is clearly demonstrated.[6] A

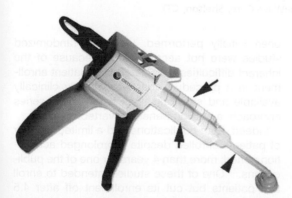

Fig. 9. Dual-chambered injection device (arrows) with bioceramic agent mixed in injection port (arrowhead) (Courtesy of Orthovita, Inc, Malvern, PA; with permission).

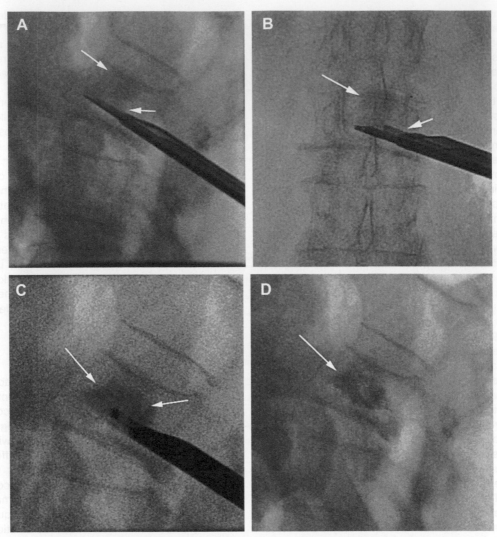

Fig. 10. Polyetheretherketone (PEEK) implants. Lateral (*A*) and frontal (*B*) radiographs of the lumbar spine showing wafer stack (*large arrows*) delivered by the surgical gun (*small arrows*) into the L2 vertebral body. A small amount of acrylic bone cement is injected around the wafer stack (*arrows*) as shown in the lateral projection (*C*) of the lumbar spine. The lateral projection of the lumbar spine (*D*) shows anterior column stabilization (*arrow*) of the L2 vertebral body with the combined implants (SpineWave Corp, Shelton, CT).

recent prospective randomized controlled trial comparing balloon-assisted vertebroplasty with conservative management showed a statistically significant difference in favor of the vertebral augmentation procedure with respect to pain relief and quality of life parameters during a 24-month period.[14] Yet, 2 recent publications with a prospective randomized controlled trial design described what was interpreted by some as "sham" therapy to be equivalent to PV for pain relief in compression fractures of the spine.[27,28] These studies would not have generated nearly as much interest if good, randomized studies of PV against conservative therapy (the traditional, historic therapy used for compression fractures before PV) had

been initially performed. However, randomized studies were not accomplished because of the inherent difficulties associated with patient enrollment in a procedure that was already clinically available and showed, albeit with a case series approach, a striking benefit to vertebroplasty.

Indeed, both publications had a limited number of patients enrolled despite a prolonged acquisition period; more than 4 years for one of the publications.[27] One of these studies intended to enroll 250 patients but cut its enrollment off after 4.5 years with 131 total patients.[29] The study reported, but did not emphasize, a trend toward a clinically meaningful improvement in pain relief for PV compared with sham therapy (64% of PV

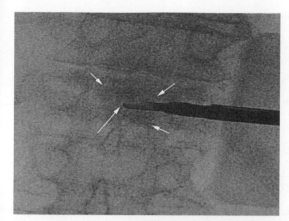

Fig. 11. Close-up view of frontal radiograph of thoracic spine showing slightly radiodense morcelized bone graft (*arrows*) being injected into acrylic mesh sac within the T12 vertebra (Spineology, St. Paul, MN).

patients vs 48% of sham-treated patients). This comparison fell short of statistical significance, with a *P* value of 0.06. Obviously, the *P* value barely missed the cutoff by 0.01 to show significance for PV to be better than the control group. Further statistical analysis of this clinical trial shows that if by continuing to enroll patients in the proportions of improved patients in each group, an additional 19 patients were needed to reach this clinical significance of PV over sham. This would have resulted in a total number of 150 patients, still far less than the intended number of 250 that was initially planned for. This simple change in the study would have nullified most of the importance as it would have shown PV to be better than sham in this category. The patient population number of 131 did not provide the sensitivity to predict this outcome.

Patients in the control group did get initial pain relief equal to PV at short-term follow-up by telephone interview. Nevertheless, it must be remembered that this sham therapy is not a conservative therapy. Actually, the sham procedure consisted of injecting an anesthetic agent into the periosteum of the fractured vertebrae (along its posterior cortex where the pedicle entry point would be if PV had been performed). On initial inspection, it might seem that this therapy should be insignificant and transient in effect; however, similar injections have been used for years in pain management. For example, facet blocks for spinal pain and occipital nerve blocks for other pains such as migraine headaches. It is not uncommon to observe the analgesic effects of these perifacet injections for weeks and sometimes months, well within the time frame of the observation period of these 2 clinical trials. Therefore, it is not surprising that

pain relief was seen with this sham procedure. Moreover, very telling is that crossover from one group to another found 43% of the sham patients crossing over to the PV group after 1 month (regardless of the amount of pain relief these patients claimed initially, it obviously did not last). Only 12% of PV patients crossed over (this is exactly expected because we find 85%–90% of patients getting good pain relief traditionally after a PV).[4] The crossover numbers were highly significant with a *P* value of 0.001.

So sham therapy was associated with initial pain relief but failed to be persistent in many treated in this group. Is this sham a real therapy or a placebo? Probably we will never know for sure, and from a clinical point of view, it may matter little. Another recent report found functional magnetic resonance imaging evidence of changes in uptake in the dorsal columns (sensory nerve region) when a placebo was applied to the skin in regions of pain.[30] This latter study shows the strong and real effect of placebo, long known to be present in most pain management treatments.

Thus, the randomized controlled trial of vertebroplasty efficacy found real or placebo effects of pain reduction with sham (not conservative) therapy. They demonstrated that the sham therapy was not long-lasting, with a statistically significant number of patients crossing over to the PV group after 1 month. Finally, if these publications had completed their initially advertised patient accrual, a clinically significant improvement in PV over sham would have been established.

CONCLUSIONS

Regardless of which of these techniques is used to perform vertebral augmentation, optimal patient outcomes are based on appropriate patient evaluation and selection. This requires appropriate clinical and imaging correlation to ascertain that there is concordance between the level of the fractured vertebra and the site and extent of the patient's symptomatology. It is, therefore, helpful to examine the patient before the procedure, under fluoroscopy when available, to determine whether the patient would potentially benefit from the procedure. The indication for a vertebral augmentation procedure is a painful, symptomatic vertebral compression fracture. Chronic vertebral compression deformities that are not painful and more recent fractures that appear to be healing and are responding to conservative management would not be indicated for treatment with this procedure under usual circumstances. Likewise, determining procedural success and optimizing patient outcomes require active patient follow-up

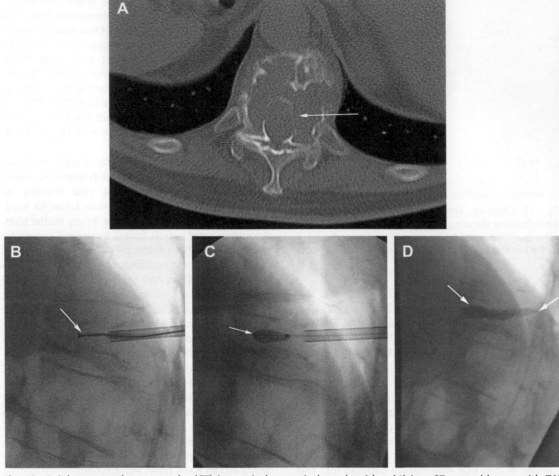

Fig. 12. Axial computed tomography (CT) image in bone window algorithm (A) in a 67-year-old man with T12 plasmacytoma shows lytic lesion with posterior cortex (arrow) destruction. Lateral radiograph of the thoracic spine (B) shows a coblation probe (arrow) inserted via coaxial technique. Lateral radiograph of the thoracic spine (C) after plasma-mediated radiofrequency ablation of the T12 lesion shows a slightly inflated balloon tamp (arrow) within the previously created cavity. Lateral radiograph of the thoracic spine (D) shows acrylic bone cement (arrows) within the vertebral body and pedicle (SpineAustin, Austin, TX).

in clinic. Elderly patients with osteoporotic vertebral compression fractures possess a myriad of potential back pain generators. Furthermore, when patients sustain a vertebral compression fracture, they also injure the adjacent supportive structures of the functional spine unit. Additional structures that might be injured during vertebral collapse include the intervertebral disk, the spinal ligaments, the facet joints, and/or the paraspinal musculature. It is therefore advisable to see, talk to, and evaluate the patients after a procedure is performed on them. Patients may claim that they still have back pain after the procedure, only to discover on examination that their pain is not a result of a failed or limited procedure but rather a result of an old pain generator such as a stenotic neural foramen or a new pain generator such as an irritated sacroiliac joint (Fig. 13). The lack of patient examination before and after the procedure is a major limitation in many of the studies that attempt to assess the efficacy of these procedures, including a recent randomized controlled trial comparing vertebroplasty with another treatment, perifacet anesthetic injections.[27] Patient follow-up allows the operator the opportunity to prescribe physical therapy along with spine rehabilitation to the patient to facilitate muscle and ligamentous healing and, most importantly, to develop good exercise and posture habits that can reduce the chances of further back injury.

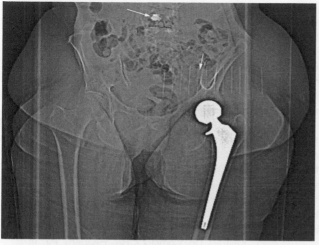 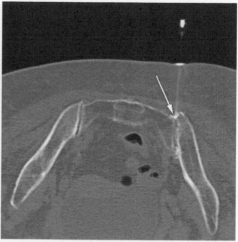

Fig. 13. Scout frontal image (*A*) from computed tomography (CT) scan of the pelvis in a patient with prior L4 vertebral augmentation (*large arrow*) shows a skin localizer grid (*small arrow*) over the left sacroiliac joint. The axial CT image in bone window algorithm (*B*) shows a 22-gauge spinal needle with its tip in the sacroiliac joint (*arrow*) and an arthrogram of the joint. The patient's sacroiliac joint pain resolved after a therapeutic injection of steroid and anesthetic.

Finally, good patient follow-up practices allow the operator the ability to initiate appropriate osteoporosis management protocols, including bone-density testing and treatment referrals, on behalf of their patients with osteoporotic vertebral compression fractures.

REFERENCES

1. Jensen ME, McGraw JK, Cardella JF, et al. Position statement on percutaneous vertebral augmentation: a consensus statement developed by the American Society of Interventional and Therapeutic Neuroradiology, Society of Interventional Radiology, American Association of Neurological Surgeons/Congress of Neurological Surgeons, and American Society of Spine Radiology. J Vasc Interv Radiol 2007;18: 325–30.

2. Galibert P, Deramond H, Rosat H, et al. [Preliminary note on the treatment of vertebral angioma by percutaneous acrylic vertebroplasty]. Neurochirurgie 1987;33:166–8 [in French].

3. Jensen ME, Evans AE, Mathis JM, et al. Percutaneous polymethylmethacrylate vertebroplasty in the treatment of osteoporotic vertebral compression fractures: technical aspects. AJNR Am J Neuroradiol 1997;18:1897–904.

4. Mathis JM, Barr JD, Belkoff SM, et al. Percutaneous vertebroplasty: a developing standard of care for vertebral compression fractures. AJNR Am J Neuroradiol 2001;22:373–81.

5. Kallmes D, Jensen ME. Percutaneous vertebroplasty. Radiology 2003;229:27–36.

6. McGirt MJ, Parker SL, Wolinsky JP, et al. Vertebroplasty and kyphoplasty for the treatment of vertebral compression fractures: and evidence-based review of the literature. Spine J 2009;9:501–8.

7. Wong W, Reiley MA, Garfin S. Vertebroplasty/kyphoplasty. J Womens Imaging 2000;2:117–24.

8. Belkoff SM, Mathis JM, Fenton DC, et al. An ex vivo biomechanical evaluation of an inflatable bone tamp used in the treatment of compression fracture. Spine 2001;26:151 6.

9. Mathis JM, Ortiz AO, Zoarski GH. Vertebroplasty versus kyphoplasty: a comparison and contrast. AJNR Am J Neuroradiol 2004;25:840–5.

10. Lieberman IH, Dudeney S, Reinhardt MK, et al. Initial outcome and efficacy of "kyphoplasty" in the treatment of painful osteoporotic vertebral compression fractures. Spine 2001;26:1631–8.

11. Phillips FM, Ho E, Campbell-Hupp M, et al. Early radiographic and clinical results of balloon kyphoplasty for the treatment of osteoporotic vertebral compression fractures. Spine 2003;28:2260–7.

12. Ortiz AO, Buonocore BJ, Zoarski GH. Height restoration following kyphoplasty for treatment of painful osteoporotoic vertebral compression fractures. J Womens Imaging 2005;7:102–10.

13. Hiwatashi A, Sidhu R, Lee RK, et al. Kyphoplasty versus vertebroplasty to increase vertebral body height: a cadaveric study. Radiology 2005;237:1115–9.

14. Wardlaw D, Cummings SR, Meirhaeghe JV, et al. Efficacy and safety of balloon kyphoplasty compared with non-surgical care for vertebral compression fracture (FREE): a randomized controlled trial. Lancet 2009;373:1016–24.

15. Brook AL, Miller TS, Fast A, et al. Vertebral augmentation with a flexible curved needle; preliminary results in 17 consecutive patients. J Vasc Interv Radiol 2008;19:1785–9.

16. Ortiz AO, Natarajan V, Gregorius D, et al. Significantly reduced radiation exposure to operators during kyphoplasty and vertebroplasty procedures: methods and techniques. AJNR Am J Neuroradiol 2006;27:989–94.

17. Georgy BA, Wong W. Plasma-mediated radiofrequency ablation assisted percutaneous cement injection for treating advanced malignant vertebral compression fractures. AJNR Am J Neuroradiol 2007;28:700–5.

18. Jasper LE, Deramond H, Mathis JM, et al. Material properties of various cements for use with vertebroplasty. J Mater Sci Mater Med 2002;14:1–5.

19. Lieberman IH, Togawa D, Kayanja MM. Vertebroplasty and kyphoplasty: filler materials. Spine J 2005;5:305S–16S.

20. Grados F, Depriester C, Cayrolle G, et al. Long-term observations of vertebral osteoporotic fractures treated by percutaneous vertebroplasty. Rheumatology(Oxford) 2000;39:1410–4.

21. Uppin AA, Hirsch JA, Centenera LV, et al. Occurrence of new vertebral body fracture after percutaneous vertebroplasty in patients with osteoporosis. Radiology 2003;226:119–24.

22. Fribourg D, Tang C, Sra P, et al. Incidence of subsequent vertebral fracture after kyphoplasty. Spine 2004;29:2270–7.

23. Harrop JS, Prpa B, Reinhardt MK, et al. Primary and secondary osteoporosis' incidence of subsequent vertebral compression fractures after kyphoplasty. Spine 2004;29:2120–5.

24. Lin EP, Ekholm S, Hiwatashi A, et al. Vertebroplasty: cement leakage into the disc increases the risk of new fracture of adjacent vertebral body. AJNR Am J Neuroradiol 2004;25:175–80.

25. Syed MI, Patel NA, Solomon J, et al. Intradiskal extravasation with low-volume cement filling in percutaneous vertebroplasty. AJNR Am J Neuroradiol 2005;26:2397–401.

26. Chiu JC, Stechison MT. Percutaneous vertebral augmentation and reconstruction with an intravertebral mesh and morcelized bone graft. Surg Technol Int 2005;14:287–96.

27. Kallmes DF, Comstock BA, Heagerty PJ, et al. A randomized trial of vertebroplasty for osteoporotic spinal fractures. N Engl J Med 2009;361:569–79.

28. Buchbinder R, Osborne RH, Ebeling PR, et al. A randomized trial of vertebroplasty for painful osteoporotic vertebral fractures. N Engl J Med 2009;361:557–68.

29. Gray LA, Jarvik JG, Heagerty PJ, et al. Investigational vertebroplasty efficacy and safety trial (INVEST): a randomized controlled trial of percutaneous vertebroplasty. BMC Blood Disord 2007;8:126–34.

30. Eippert F, Finsterbusch J, Bingel U, et al. Direct evidence for spinal cord involvement in placebo analgesia. Science 2009;326:404.

Biomechanics of Vertebral Bone Augmentation

Celene Hadley, MD[a], Omer Abdulrehman Awan, MD[a],
Gregg H. Zoarski, MD[b],*

KEYWORDS

- Vertebral augmentation • Vertebroplasty • Kyphoplasty
- Biomechanics • Kyphosis

The primary goal of percutaneous vertebral augmentation is to provide relief from vertebrogenic pain associated with a pathologic compression fracture or marrow infiltration. These processes may be related to either primary or secondary osteoporosis or benign or malignant neoplasm. Percutaneous vertebral augmentation may prevent further collapse of the fractured vertebral body, which leads to further loss of height, fractures at adjacent levels, and progressive kyphosis. In addition, patients with vertebral compression fracture have a 23% to 34% increase in mortality rate compared with patients without fracture; the most common cause of death in these patients is pulmonary disease, including chronic obstructive pulmonary disease and pneumonia.[1]

Percutaneous vertebral augmentation is a successful means of relieving pain and reducing disability after vertebral compression fracture[2]; however, the exact mechanism by which vertebral augmentation eliminates pain remains unproven. Most likely, pain relief is due to stabilization of microfractures. The biomechanical effects of vertebral fracture and subsequent vertebral augmentation therapy, however, are topics for continued investigation. Altered biomechanical stresses after treatment may affect the risk of adjacent fracture in an osteoporotic patient; that risk may be different after vertebral augmentation with cavity creation (balloon assisted vertebroplasty or kyphoplasty) versus vertebral augmentation without cavity creation (vertebroplasty). Polymethyl methacrylate (PMMA) cement used in these procedures may have an important effect on the load transfer and disk mechanics, and therefore, the variables of cement volume, formulation, and distribution should also be evaluated. Finally, the question of whether prophylactic treatment of adjacent intact levels is indicated must be considered.

BIOMECHANICS

A fundamental understanding of the regional biomechanics is essential when considering the osteoporotic spine and the effects of vertebral augmentation. Under physiologic conditions, load is shared by the vertebrae, disks, ligaments, facet joints, and, in the thoracic region, the ribs and sternum. Compressive load is generated by the weight of the body segments and the action of the trunk muscles. When devising experimental models of the spine, preservation of these nonosseous components is essential for the validity of some ex vivo models. Experimental models that study a functional unit of the spine comprising multiple vertebral body levels and their supporting structures may therefore be most relevant.

Two major factors likely contribute to anterior vertebral body stress and increased potential for adjacent level fractures after an initial vertebral compression fracture: anterior load shift and changes in load transfer through the intervertebral disk. Kyphosis from a vertebral compression fracture causes an anterior shift of the compressive load path in the fractured as well as the adjacent

a University of Maryland Medical Center, 22 South Greene Street, Baltimore, MD 21201, USA
b Division of Neurosciences, University of Maryland Medical Center, 22 South Greene Street, Baltimore, MD 21201, USA
* Corresponding author.
E-mail address: gzoarski@umm.edu

Neuroimag Clin N Am 20 (2010) 159–167
doi:10.1016/j.nic.2010.02.002

unfractured vertebral bodies by increasing the moment arm.[3] In an osteoporotic vertebral body, this can increase peak stresses by up to 2.5 times. With endplate fracture, load transfer through the disk is altered as the volume of space occupied by the nucleus pulposus increases; the nucleus is then unable to increase pressure during flexion. Because of this loss of a cushion effect, the anterior annulus and apophyseal ring bear more load stress during flexion, potentially leading to increased risk of adjacent level fracture.[4]

If the increasing kyphosis increases the risk of additional fractures, one might assume that reducing or preventing the worsening kyphosis may be beneficial. To determine the effect of thoracic vertebral compression fractures on kyphosis or on geometric alignment and shift of load path alignment, Gaitanis and colleagues[4] performed a biomechanical study using human thoracic specimens. These specimens were also used to evaluate geometric and load path alignment after fracture reduction by balloon bone tamp and by spinal extension alone. Six fresh thoracic specimens of 3 adjacent vertebrae with intact adjacent soft tissues (a functional spine unit) were used as the model. In this study, the compressive load shifted anteriorly by 7.8 mm after a single fracture of the middle of the 3 vertebral elements or by 22% of the anteroposterior dimension of the endplate of the fractured vertebra. The supraadjacent vertebra demonstrated a 23% shift (7.9 mm), and the subjacent vertebra demonstrated an 18% shift (6.4 mm). After treatment of the fractured vertebra using a bone tamp, segmental kyphosis was corrected by 8.7° (66%) and vertebral kyphosis was corrected by 11° (85%). Although the load path was returned more posteriorly, it remained anterior to the prefracture load path; 56% of the postfracture change was recovered.

In the same study, cementation with only hyperextension corrected anterior vertebral deformity to near prefracture values; however, segmental kyphosis and middle height were not corrected. The investigators concluded that bone tamp inflation significantly reduced deformity of the vertebral body height and kyphosis and resulted in return of the load path to near prefracture alignment. Hyperextension alone improved vertebral body deformity and load path alignment, without restoring middle vertebral height and kyphotic deformity.[4]

Correction of kyphosis of the fractured vertebral body does not necessarily correlate with overall kyphosis correction. Pradhan and colleagues[5] performed a retrospective study of 65 patients who had undergone 1 to 3 level kyphoplasty, analyzing the pre- and postoperative radiographs.

Height gain was maximal at the midvertebral body (39%, 6.4 mm) and less in the anterior vertebral body (15%, 3.1 mm). For single level kyphoplasty, vertebral kyphosis was reduced by 7.3°. However, segmental kyphotic deformity was reduced by only 2.4° at 1 level, 1.4° at 2 levels, and 1° at 3 levels above and below the treated vertebra. Most kyphosis correction obtained in this study was limited to the treated vertebral body; a phenomenon which the investigators suggested may be attributable to the absorptive properties of the intervertebral disk.[5]

RISK OF ADJACENT FRACTURE

Adjacent level fractures certainly occur after vertebral augmentation; however, because the natural history of osteoporosis also demonstrates a high fracture rate in the same load-bearing zone, the cause of adjacent level fracture may not be easily ascertained.

It is generally accepted that 20% of patients who suffer an initial vertebral compression fracture and are not treated with systemic osteoporosis therapy experience an additional vertebral compression fracture within 1 year. It is difficult to discriminate between the effect of vertebral augmentation and the powerful influence of natural history. The presence of a single osteoporotic vertebral compression fracture increases the risk of a new fracture by at least 5-fold. The presence of 2 or more osteoporotic vertebral compression fractures at baseline increases the risk of a new fracture by 12 times.[6] According to the literature, the risk of new adjacent fractures with vertebroplasty ranges from 0% to 16%.[7–13] For kyphoplasty, the risk ranges from 45% to 75% (Fig. 1).[14–17]

Studies on percutaneous vertebral augmentation to date have not stratified patients based on the extent and severity of osteoporosis. Many patients who present for percutaneous vertebral fracture reduction are not being managed for osteoporosis. Existing studies on percutaneous vertebral augmentation have not included the effect of posttreatment management, including bisphosphonates and physical therapy. In the setting of osteoporosis, the incidence of subsequent vertebral compression fracture may decrease after the initiation of bisphosphonate therapy.

In a study with 1-year follow-up, 24% of the patients (16 out of 66) treated with percutaneous vertebroplasty developed new compression fractures (a total of 26 new fractures). Half of these new fractures were adjacent to the treated vertebral bodies; however, the presence of more than 2 preexisting compression fractures was found

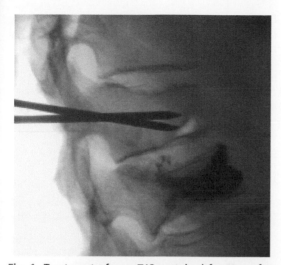

Fig. 1. Treatment of new T12 vertebral fracture after prior L1 vertebroplasty. Adjacent level fractures certainly occur after vertebral augmentation; however, because the natural history of osteoporosis also predicts a high fracture rate in the same load-bearing zone, the cause of adjacent level fracture may not be easily ascertained.

to be the only independent risk factor for developing a new compression fracture.[18]

In a prospective study of 25 patients with 34 fractures who were treated with percutaneous vertebroplasty and followed for 48 months, 13 patients (52%) developed at least 1 new vertebral fracture during follow-up. The odds ratio for a new compression fracture in the vicinity of a treated vertebra was 2.27 compared with 1.44 for a new fracture in the vicinity of an untreated vertebra and was not statistically significant.[19]

To further complicate the analysis, patients with primary and secondary osteoporosis may have a different incidence of fracture after kyphoplasty than patients with primary osteoporosis. In a retrospective review, 22.6% of patients (26 of 115) demonstrated new compression fractures after kyphoplasty. Thirty-five percent of these patients had primary osteoporosis and 17% had steroid induced osteoporosis. The incidence of postkyphoplasty fracture was 11.25% (9 out of 80) in patients with primary osteoporosis. In contrast, the incidence of postkyphoplasty fracture in patients with secondary osteoporosis was 48.6% (17 out of 35), a statistically significant increase.[14]

Mudano and colleagues performed a retrospective study to compare the risk of subsequent fracture in patients with an initially treated versus untreated vertebral compression fracture over 18 months. New compression fractures were defined as occurring 90 to 360 days after the index event and at a different level than the baseline fracture.

Of the 48 treated patients, 51% had undergone vertebroplasty and 49% had undergone kyphoplasty. Information on bisphosphonate therapy was lacking. Risk of a subsequent fracture at a new level within 90 days was 5 times greater in treated patients than in the untreated comparison group. Incidence of subsequent vertebral compression fractures doubled at 360 days, by 18.8% in the treated group and 9.7% in the comparison group. At 360 days after the index fracture, 19% of treated patients had subsequent compression fractures compared with only 7% in the comparison group. Median time to new fracture was 2 months in the treatment group versus 3 months in the control group. All new fractures occurred within 3 levels of the index fracture.[20] Fracture incidence after vertebroplasty and kyphoplasty were not compared.

Multiple studies have reported the incidence of subsequent fractures after vertebroplasty or kyphoplasty; extremely variable results may reflect the complexity of factors involved. In a retrospective review of 177 patients treated with percutaneous vertebroplasty over 2 years, 12.4% (22 patients) were found to have a total of 36 new compression fractures. Of these, 67%[21] of the fractures occurred adjacent to previously treated vertebrae, and 33% (12) occurred in nonadjacent vertebrae. Of the 36 new compression fractures, 67%[21] occurred within 30 days of initial treatment. It is important to note that this study involved a bipedicular approach in 60 (86%) of the 70 vertebroplasties performed, using an average of 9.14 mL of PMMA (ranging from 5–14.5 mL).[9] In another study, 12.5% (3 out of 23) of treated patients experienced additional fractures at untreated levels within 15 to 18 months of vertebroplasty.[2] In a retrospective review of patients treated with kyphoplasty, 26% (10 out of 38 patients) sustained new compression fractures over an average of 8-month follow-up.[15]

Increased risk of adjacent level fracture in kyphoplasty as compared with vertebroplasty has been reported by Frankel, whose study included 36 patients with 46 compression fractures. Kyphoplasty was performed in 17 patients with 20 compression fractures, using an average of 4.65 mL cement. Ninety-five percent of the procedures were bilateral and 15% demonstrated cement extravasation. Vertebroplasty was performed in 19 patients with a total of 26 compression fractures, using an average of 3.78 mL cement. Nineteen percent of the procedures were bilateral with 7.7% cement extravasation. Pain improved in 90% of both groups. Within 90 days, 5 new adjacent fractures were seen in patients treated with kyphoplasty, whereas no new adjacent fractures were seen in those treated with vertebroplasty. The investigators concluded that vertebroplasty offers comparable pain relief with less cement and a unilateral approach and with significantly less risk of adjacent fracture.[21]

THE ROLE OF CEMENT

The role of cement includes eliminating pain, restoring biomechanical strength and stiffness, maintaining intraoperative and postoperative fracture reduction, and preventing refracture. Variability in distribution, amount, formulation, and subsequent load transfer may have an effect on all of these functions. Posttreatment vertebral body strength can be variable and may be restored to prefracture strength or even to a healthy, normal value. But because the stiffness of PMMA cements may be significantly more than that of osteoporotic bone, the effect of PMMA on overall spine stiffness and intervertebral disk stiffness warrants consideration.

Strain is a measure of deformation of the material to which forces are being applied. Different types of strain include compressive, tensile, and shear strain. Compressive strain is the ratio of contraction of the material to its original length, tensile strain is the ratio of elongation of a material to its original length, and shear strain is the ratio of deflection of the material, in the direction of the shear force, and the distance between shear forces. Consider a rod with an initial length of L that is stretched to a length L'. The tensile strain measure (ϵ) is a dimensionless value and is defined as the ratio of elongation with respect to the original length. Stiffness (K), on the other hand, is defined as the ratio of an applied force (P) over the distance (d) that a body deflects in response to that force. Elastic modulus is not the same as stiffness, whereas stiffness depends on the material, including the shape and the boundary conditions; elastic modulus is a property of the constituent material alone. The literature varies widely in reports of posttreatment vertebral body stiffness, possibly due to the differences among models used for experimentation. In particular, the use of isolated vertebral segments, functional spine units, and the presence or absence of supporting soft tissue structures may affect the outcome of studies on this subject (**Figs. 2** and **3**).

With percutaneous vertebroplasty, vertebral body strength can be restored after injection of only 2 mL of cement; however, restoration of stiffness requires 4 mL in the thoracic spine, 4 to 8 mL in the thoracolumbar spine (depending on the type of cement used), and 4 to 6 mL in the lumbar spine.[22] It is important to note that in the thoracic

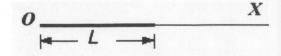

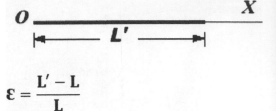

$$\varepsilon = \frac{L' - L}{L}$$

$$k = \frac{P}{d}$$

Fig. 2. A metal rod of length (L) is stretched to a length (L'). The tensile strain (ϵ) is defined as the ratio of elongation with respect to the original length. Stiffness (K) is defined by the ratio of an applied force (P) over the distance (d) that an object deflects in response to the applied force.

spine as little as 2 mL of cement can provide pain relief.[23] Use of lower cement volumes may decrease the risk of complications, including cement extravasation, and possibly reduce strain at adjacent levels.

In addition to the amount of cement injected, posttreatment strength may be strongly dependent on endplate-to-endplate filling. In a study comparing 35% and 25% fracture groups, the 35% fracture group's posttreatment strength was significantly less when cement did not span endplate to endplate (767 vs 1141 N). The posttreatment strength was 106% of the initial vertebral body strength in the endplate-to-endplate group when compared with 65% in the partial treatment group. Steens and colleagues concluded that endplate-to-endplate augmentation is desirable, providing for better postoperative strength, and that "safe volumes" as recommended by some authorities to avoid complications do not likely result in endplate-to-endplate filling. Because no difference in vertebral body strength was observed in the 25% fracture group posttreatment compared with the untreated vertebrae group, the investigators concluded that vertebral fracture models with 25% deformation are unsuitable to assess the biomechanical effects of vertebral augmentation (**Fig. 4**).[24]

In another study, isolated osteoporotic cadaveric vertebrae were subjected to compression

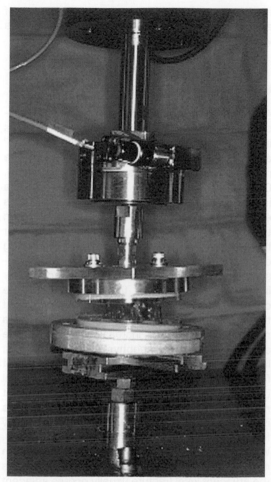

Fig. 3. An Instron device (Instron Worldwide Head-quarters, Norwood, MA, USA) can be used to evaluate the mechanical properties of vertebral bodies in compression experiments.

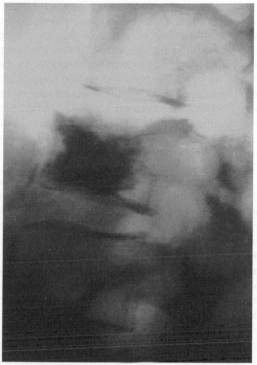

Fig. 4. Endplate-to-endplate vertebral filling after cement injection. In addition to the amount and type of cement injected, posttreatment strength may be strongly dependent on endplate-to-endplate filling.

loading before and after infiltration with acrylic bone cement. Although the cemented specimen did not completely adopt the properties of bulk bone cement, the effect of cement infiltration on cancellous bone was considerable, with stiffness measuring 8.5 times than that of native bone. The local stiffening of cancellous bone in the treated vertebrae may alter the load transfer of the augmented motion segment, a possible cause of subsequent fractures in vertebrae adjacent to those infiltrated with cement.[25]

Boger and colleagues[26] performed a biomechanical study of low-modulus cement to determine the effect of PMMA formulation on adjacent fractures. The goal of the study was to determine whether or not low-modulus PMMA decreases the likelihood of adjacent fractures in clinical and experimental studies. This model used functional spine units of nonfractured T9-L4 vertebrae, 92% of which were osteoporotic. All soft tissues were dissected with preservation of ligaments and facet capsules. There were 3 groups: untreated, those treated with low-modulus PMMA, and those treated with regular PMMA. Low-modulus cement had been previously characterized as having similar mechanical properties as cancellous bone in compression.[27] Cement filling extended from upper to lower endplates. Results were limited to prophylactic vertebroplasty but demonstrated no difference in overall spinal stiffness and no significant reduction in failure rate with low-modulus PMMA when compared with controls. A higher incidence of adjacent endplate fractures occurred at lower loads with regular PMMA than with controls. With low-modulus PMMA, adjacent fractures were evenly distributed above and below the treated level. With regular PMMA, adjacent fractures occurred above the treated level in 10 out of 11 times.[26]

Finite element analysis solves partial differential equations over complex domains when the domain changes (eg, a crash test simulation), and it is a suitable method for addressing questions about elastic and structural analysis. Finite element analysis has been used to evaluate the effect of cement augmentation on load transfer; increased pressure in the nucleus pulposus and bulge of the adjacent endplate are associated with increased stresses and strains in the vertebrae next to an augmentation. Changes to the overall stress and strain distribution were found to be less pronounced for unipedicular augmentation.[28] From these findings it was concluded that the treatment clearly altered load transfer, ultimately supporting the hypothesis that rigid cement augmentation may facilitate the subsequent collapse of adjacent vertebrae (**Fig. 5**).[28]

Rohlmann and colleagues[29] used a model of the lumbar spine to estimate the forces of the trunk muscles, the intradiskal pressure, and the stresses in the endplates in the intact spine before and after vertebroplasty and kyphoplasty. The results demonstrated that when a wedge-shaped fracture occurs, the upper body moves anteriorly, requiring higher forces at the erector spinae muscles to maintain equilibrium at the thoracolumbar junction. These forces were increased by 200%, even after vertebroplasty. In addition, vertebral fracture results in increased intradiskal pressures of 15% to 22% when compared with an intact spine. Intradiskal pressures, however, increased only minimally after cement injection. Thus, adjacent fractures were felt to be more likely the result of increased load rather than increased stiffness. It was concluded that although cement augmentation alone provides stabilization and pain relief, it does not improve spinal alignment, restore disk biomechanics, or restore prefracture load transfer. Also, the correction of spinal deformity and load

alignment can provide benefit; the correction of endplate deformity and load transfer may also be very important.[29]

BIOMECHANICS OF INTERVERTEBRAL DISKS

Although intradiskal pressure may not be significantly increased after cement injection, it is increased after vertebral compression fracture,[29] and the role of altered disk biomechanics in the risk of adjacent fractures must be considered. During normal flexion, intradiskal pressure increases along with increasing load. This load is evenly distributed as the strain increases. When the endplate fractures, the space available for the nucleus pulposus is increased; increasing disk volume results in diminished intradiskal pressure. When the nuclear pressure no longer increases during flexion, there is a loss of the cushion effect; load is distributed to the rim of the disk and the strain doubles. The annulus bears more weight and strain, increasing the load on the anterior portion of the apophyseal ring with flexion, leading to increased risk of subsequent adjacent fractures.[30,31] After cement fixation, the vertebral body is filled with PMMA and the vertebral height may be restored; however, the endplate fracture is not necessarily reduced and space available for the nucleus pulposus may remain increased. With flexion, the disk pressure is still lower than normal and the anterior stress still doubles, thus the adjacent level fracture usually occurs adjacent to the fractured endplate.[30]

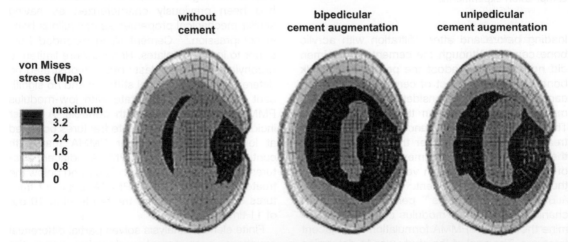

Fig. 5. von Mises stress distribution in the L2 inferior endplate (caudal view) for an osteoporotic functional spinal unit resulting from 1000 N of compression. Stress distribution if no filling was simulated (*left*). Stress distribution if L3 received bipedicular PMMA filling (*middle*). Distribution for a unipedicular augmentation of L3 (*right*). (*Reprinted from* Polikeit A, Nolte LP, Ferguson SJ. The effect of cement augmentation on the load transfer in an osteoporotic functional spinal unit: finite-element analysis. Spine (Phila Pa 1976) 2003;28(10):994; with permission.)

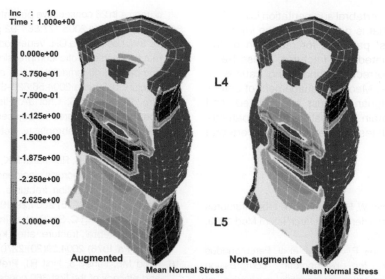

Fig. 6. A comparison of stresses in a motion segment, showing the load shift that results from the rigid cement augmentation. The colors represent the mean stresses (MPa) in the sagittal plane in response to a quasi-static compression. In the nonaugmented motion segment (*right*), the endplates bulge symmetrically (*green*) in response to nucleus hydrostatic pressure (*blue*), subjecting the adjacent cancellous bone to symmetric compressive stresses in the range of 1 to 1.5 MPa (*green*). In the augmented motion segment (*left*), the augmented cancellous bone of the L5 vertebral body (lower) acts as a pillar supporting the endplate. As a result, the forces are transmitted to cancellous bone by compression (*light green*) as opposed to the bending (bulge) in the nonaugmented bone. In response to the decreased bulge of the L5 superior endplate, the nuclear pressure increases (*blue*). As a result, the bulge of the inferior L4 endplate and the compressive stress in the L4 cancellous bone (*dark green*) increase by approximately 17%. (*Reprinted from* Baroud G, Nemes J, Heini P, et al. Load shift of the intervertebral disc after a vertebroplasty: a finite-element study. Eur Spine J 2003;12:423; with permission.)

Baroud and colleagues used a finite element model of a lumbar motion segment (L4-5) to quantify and compare the pre- and postaugmentation stiffness and loading of the intervertebral disk adjacent to the augmented vertebra in static compression. The bulge of the augmented endplate was reduced to 7% of its value before the augmentation, resulting in a stiffening of the intervertebral joint by approximately 17% and of the whole motion segment by approximately 11%. The intervertebral pressure increased accordingly by 19%, and the inward bulge of the endplate adjacent to the augmented vertebra increased considerably by approximately 17%. It was concluded that this increase of 17% may be the cause of the adjacent posttreatment fractures, with the rigid cement augmentation underneath the endplates acting as an upright pillar, severely reducing the inward bulge of the endplates of the augmented vertebra (**Fig. 6**).[32]

PROPHYLAXIS

Hypothetical advantages of prophylactic vertebral fracture augmentation with PMMA include retention of normal vertebral body height, retention of normal alignment, and reduced risk of cement leakage.[33] Thus far, however, there has been considerable speculation on both sides of the debate but little if any scientific investigation. Any conclusions that are drawn about prophylaxis are currently based on extrapolation from existing literature rather than on directed investigation. Furthermore, existing and future bioactive materials may be more suitable to prophylaxis than PMMA.

SUMMARY

Vertebral body compression fractures alter load alignment and the function of the intervertebral disk. Kyphosis correction at 1 or even 2 adjacent levels fails to achieve significant sagittal realignment or kyphosis correction. The incidence of adjacent fractures after percutaneous vertebral augmentation may be higher than without treatment and may be even higher still with kyphoplasty. Vertebropasty offers comparable pain relief with less cement than kyphoplasty and a unilateral approach, with apparently less risk of adjacent fracture. Adjacent fractures are related to multiple factors but may be more likely due to the resultant increased load and geometric misalignment rather than increased stiffness.

Percutaneous vertebral augmentation is a palliative procedure that is performed for the improvement of patients' pain and for reduction of the morbidity associated with fractures. These treatments do no correct the underlying causes of vertebral fracture. Medical management of osteoporosis or malignancy must be initiated and continued to obtain maximal benefit in patients who are candidates for percutaneous vertebral fracture repair.

REFERENCES

1. Kado D, Browner W, Palmermo L. Vertebral fractures and mortality in older women. Arch Intern Med 1999; 159(11):1215–20.
2. Zoarski GH, Snow P, Olan WJ, et al. Percutaneous vertebroplasty for osteoporotic compression fractures: quantitative prospective evaluation of long-term outcomes. J Vasc Interv Radiol 2002; 13(2 Pt 1):139–48.
3. Yuan H, Brown C, Phillips F. Osteoporotic spinal deformity a biomechanical rationale for the clinical consequences and treatment of vertebral body compression fractures. J Spinal Disord Tech 2004; 17(3):236–42.
4. Gaitanis IN, Carandang G, Phillips FM, et al. Restoring geometric and loading alignment of the thoracic spine with a vertebral compression fracture: effects of balloon (bone tamp) inflation and spinal extension. Spine J 2005;5(1):45–54.
5. Pradhan BB, Bae HW, Kropf MA, et al. Kyphoplasty reduction of osteoporotic vertebral compression fractures: correction of local kyphosis versus overall sagittal alignment. Spine (Phila Pa 1976) 2006;31(4): 435–41.
6. Ross PD, Davis JW, Epstein RS. Pre-existing fractures and bone mass predict vertebral fracture incidence in women. Ann Intern Med 1991;113:919–23.
7. Peh WC, Gilula LA, Peck DD. Percutaneous vertebroplasty for severe osteoporotic vertebral body compression fractures. Radiology 2002;223:121–6.
8. Syed MI, Patel NA, Jan S. Intradiskal extravasation with low-volume cement filling in percutaneous vertebroplasty. AJNR Am J Neuroradiol 2005;26: 2397–401.
9. Uppin AA, Hirsch JA, Centenera LV, et al. Occurrence of new vertebral body fracture after percutaneous vertebroplasty in patients with osteoporosis. Radiology 2003;226(1):119–24.
10. Tanigawa N, Komemushi A, Kariya S. Radiological follow-up of new compression fractures following percutaneous vertebroplasty. Cardiovasc Intervent Radiol 2005;29:92–6.
11. Fessl R, Roemer FW, Bohndorf K. [Percutaneous vertebroplasty for the osteoporotic vertebral compression fractures: experiences and prospective clinical

outcome in 26 consecutive patients with 50 vertebral fractures]. Rofo 2005;177:884–92 [in German].
12. Yu SW, Lee PC, Ma CH. Vertebroplasty for the treatment of osteoporotic compression spinal fracture: comparison of remedial action at different stages of injury. J Trauma 2004;56:629–32.
13. Kim SH, Kang HS, Choi JA. Risk factors of new compression fractures in adjacent vertebrae after percutaneous vertebroplasty. Acta Radiol 2004;45: 440–5.
14. Harrop JS, Prpa B, Reinhardt MK, et al. Primary and secondary osteoporosis' incidence of subsequent vertebral compression fractures after kyphoplasty. Spine (Phila Pa 1976) 2004;29(19):2120–5.
15. Fribourg D, Tang C, Sra P, et al. Incidence of subsequent vertebral fracture after kyphoplasty. Spine (Phila Pa 1976) 2004;29(20):2270–6.
16. Majd ME, Farley S, Holt RT. Preliminary outcomes and efficacy of the first 360 consecutive kyphoplasties for the treatment of painful osteoporotic vertebral compression fractures. Spine J 2005;5:244–55.
17. Gaitanis IN, Hadjipavlou AG, Katonis PG. Balloon kyphoplasty for the treatment of pathological vertebral compressive fractures. Eur Spine J 2004;14: 250–60.
18. Voormolen MH, Lohle PN, Juttmann JR, et al. The risk of new osteoporotic vertebral compression fractures in the year after percutaneous vertebroplasty. J Vasc Interv Radiol 2006;17(1):71–6.
19. Grados F, Depriester C, Cayrolle G, et al. Long-term observations of vertebral osteoporotic fractures treated by percutaneous vertebroplasty. Rheumatology (Oxford) 2000;39(12):1410–4.
20. Mudano AS, Bian J, Cope JU, et al. Vertebroplasty and kyphoplasty are associated with an increased risk of secondary vertebral compression fractures: a population-based cohort study. Osteoporos Int 2009;20(5):819–26.
21. Frankel BM, Monroe T, Wang C. Percutaneous vertebral augmentation: an elevation in adjacent-level fracture risk in kyphoplasty as compared with vertebroplasty. Spine J 2007;7(5):575–82.
22. Belkoff S, Mathis J, Jasper L, et al. The biomechanics of vertebroplasty: the effect of cement volume on mechanical behavior. Spine (Phila Pa 1976) 2001;26(14):1537–41.
23. Cotton A, Dewatre F, Cortet B, et al. Percutaneous vertebroplasty for osteolytic metastases and myeloma; effects of the percentage of lesion filling and the leakage of methyl methacrylate at clinical follow-up. Radiology 1996;200:525–30.
24. Steens J, Verdonschot N, Aalsma AM, et al. The influence of endplate-to-endplate cement augmentation on vertebral strength and stiffness in vertebroplasty. Spine (Phila Pa 1976) 2007;32(15):E419–22.
25. Baroud G, Nemes J, Ferguson SJ, et al. Material changes in osteoporotic human cancellous bone

following infiltration with acrylic bone cement for a vertebral cement augmentation. Comput Methods Biomech Biomed Engin 2003;6(2):133–9.

26. Boger A, Heini P, Windolf M, et al. Adjacent vertebral failure after vertebroplasty: a biomechanical study of low-modulus PMMA cement. Eur Spine J 2007; 16(12):2118–25.

27. Boger A, Bohner M, Heini P, et al. Properties of a low-modulus PMMA bone cement for osteoporotic bone. Eur Cell Mater 2005;10(1):17.

28. Polikeit A, Nolte LP, Ferguson SJ. The effect of cement augmentation on the load transfer in an osteoporotic functional spinal unit: finite-element analysis. Spine (Phila Pa 1976) 2003;28(10):991–6.

29. Rohlmann A, Zander T, Bergmann G. Spinal loads after osteoporotic vertebral fractures treated by vertebroplasty or kyphoplasty. Eur Spine J 2006;15(8): 1255–64.

30. Tzermiadianos MN, Renner SM, Havey R, et al. Decreased disc pressure after a vertebral endplate fracture. Is it an additional risk factor for fractures at the adjacent levels? Presented at 53rd Annual Orthopaedic Research Society Meeting. San Diego, CA, February 11–14, 2007. Poster 1028.

31. Tzermiadianos MN, Renner SM, Phillips FM, et al. Altered disc pressure profile after an osteoporotic vertebral fracture is a risk factor for adjacent vertebral body fracture. Eur Spine J 2008;17(11): 1522–30.

32. Baroud G, Heini P, Nemes J, et al. Biomechanical explanation of adjacent fractures following vertebroplasty. Radiology 2003;229:606–7.

33. Becker S, Garoscio M, Meissner J, et al. Is there an indication for prophylactic balloon kyphoplasty? A pilot study. Clin Orthop Relat Res 2007;458: 83–9.

Vertebroplasty Technique in Metastatic Disease

Bassem A. Georgy, MD[a,b,*]

KEYWORDS

• Vertebroplasty • Kyphoplasty • Metastasis

Metastatic bone tumors in the spine are painful and debilitating but are challenging to treat. Percutaneous approaches for performing vertebral body augmentation for treating metastatic spinal lesions have been developed as good alternatives to open surgery and for pain control. These types of procedures have evolved rapidly during the last 10 years, and the current state of the art has been found to fit neatly into the conventional oncologic treatment algorithm.

EPIDEMIOLOGY AND CLINICAL PRESENTATION

Spinal metastasis is the most commonly encountered tumor of the spine,[1] occurring in up to 40% of patients with cancer.[2] Each year, 5% of patients with cancer, or approximately 61,000 persons, develop spinal metastasis.[3] The cancers most often metastasizing to the spine include breast (21%), lung (14%), prostate (8%), renal (5%), gastrointestinal (5%), and thyroid (3%) cancers. The posterior half of the vertebral body is usually infiltrated first, with the anterior body, lamina, and pedicles becoming involved later.[4] The treatment regimen for spinal metastasis is generally palliative and consists of a combination of medical therapy (steroids, pain medication, and chemotherapy), radiation therapy, and surgery.

When managing patients affected by spinal metastasis, the primary goals of treatment are to relieve pain and preserve or restore function.

Pain is generally described in at least 1 of 3 ways:

1. Constant and localized
2. Radicular
3. Axial, coinciding with functional disability.

Localized pain is generally thought to be a result of periosteal stretch occurring with tumor expansion and is usually treated using radiation because this therapy is effective for decreasing the tumor size. Radicular pain, most likely caused by the tumor pressing against the nerve root, is also addressed using radiation therapy but can be treated using nerve root blocks as well. Axial pain, most frequently associated with mechanical instability of the spine or pathologic vertebral body fracture, is worsened with physical activity but relieved with rest. Axial pain has been traditionally treated by surgically stabilizing the spine.

BIOMECHANICS OF PATHOLOGIC FRACTURES

In patients with spinal metastasis, pathologic fracture can occur under normal physiologic stress.[5] Partial or total destruction of the anterior vertebral body results in decreased load-bearing capacity of the spine. How and when pathologic fracture occurs is generally determined by the size and location of the tumor, the extent of tumor destruction, and the patient's bone mineral density.[1,6] Ventrally situated tumors (anterior column) have a potentially greater destabilizing effect than

Disclosures: Consultant, Arthrocare Spine, Inc, DePuy Spine, Inc, and Dfine, Inc; Member Advisory Board and shareholder, Spine Align, Osseon Therapeutics LLC.
[a] North County Radiology, 488 East Valley Parkway, Suite 214, Escondido, CA 92025, USA
[b] Department of Radiology, University of California, San Diego, 200 West Arbor Drive, San Diego, CA 92103, USA
* North County Radiology, 488 East Valley Parkway, Suite 214, Escondido, CA 92025.
E-mail address: bassemgeorgy@ymail.com

Neuroimag Clin N Am 20 (2010) 169–177
doi:10.1016/j.nic.2010.02.003

dorsally located masses (middle column) in the presence of intact dorsal elements.[7]

THE CONVENTIONAL TREATMENT REGIMEN
Radiation Therapy

Radiotherapy has a long history of proven success for alleviating pain in patients with metastatic spinal lesions when they are radiosensitive. Earlier studies evaluating the success of radiation therapy showed that neurologic improvement was obtained in 40% to 50% of patients, but more recent studies have demonstrated a success rate of 70%.[8,9] Pain relief may be delayed for up to 2 weeks after the start of radiotherapy,[10] and this treatment does not correct existing biomechanical abnormalities or stabilize the spine. In addition, it is not effective for preventing imminent vertebral body collapse; almost half of the patients undergoing radiotherapy subsequently experience vertebral body compression fractures.[11,12] Because of these drawbacks, adding a spine stabilization procedure to a radiation therapy program is thought to be critical for rapidly managing axial pain and for providing neurologic recovery.[13,14]

Open Surgery

Historically, the indications for surgical intervention have included radioresistant disease, spinal instability, spinal cord compression, acute or progressive neurologic deterioration, previous exposure of the spinal cord to radiation, incapacitating pain (despite orthotic treatment or radiation), impending pathologic fracture, and life expectancy of at least 3 months.[14] The principal objectives of surgery include nerve root decompression, stabilization, and reconstruction of the anatomic spinal column.[2] Surgery is thought to maximize the patient's quality of life because it is likely to restore or preserve neurologic function and relieve pain. Nevertheless, prospective surgical candidates must be considered adequately fit for undergoing a surgical

procedure that is associated with high risk of significant complications.

The surgical approach depends on

1. Location of the tumor
2. Presence or absence of spinal instability and
3. Presence or absence of neural compression or neural deficit.

In 1989, Weinstein[15] proposed a model designed to enhance surgical planning in patients with spinal metastasis. In this model, the vertebral body is delineated into 4 zones (**Fig. 1**), which are used to describe location of the metastatic lesion. Zone I includes the spinous process to pars interarticularis and superior facet. Zone II encompasses the superior articular facet, transverse process, and the pedicle from the level of the pars to its junction with the vertebral body. Zone III consists of the anterior three-quarters of the vertebral body, and zone IV is the posterior one-quarter of the vertebral body. Within these zones, the tumor itself is described as intraosseous, extraosseous, or distance metastasis.

Zone I and zone II lesions are accessed using a posterior or posterolateral surgical approach. These types of lesions are usually treated using posterior decompression and stabilization. Zone III lesions are typically accessed using an anterior surgical approach; this allows direct access to the tumor, and effective reconstruction of the weight-bearing anterior portion of the spinal column can be achieved using allograft, autograft, cages, plates, or polymethylmethacrylate implants.[14] Zone IV lesions are the most difficult to treat because they require a combined anterior and posterior approach.

PERCUTANEOUS IMAGE-GUIDED VERTEBRAL BODY AUGMENTATION

In 1981, Harrington[16] was the first to propose using bone cement augmentation as a method for relieving pain that is associated with malignant

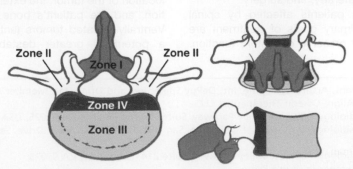

Fig. 1. The vertebral body and adjacent structures can be depicted as 4 disparate zones when considering surgery to treat vertebral body tumors.

spinal tumors. In essence, the investigator described a "fusion" type of procedure, in which bone cement was inserted around and into tumor-affected vertebral bodies after removing portions of the tumor, as a method to stabilize the spine.

Subsequently, percutaneous vertebral body augmentation procedures, such as vertebroplasty and kyphoplasty, were developed as a means for managing malignant spine lesions and used with good success. During the mid-1990s, Cotten and colleagues[17] reported that 97% of patients had at least some pain relief within the first 48 hours after undergoing a vertebroplasty procedure. Of these patients, 13.5% were pain free, 55% showed substantial improvement, and 30% were moderately improved (Fig. 2). Weill and colleageus[18] reported that 73% and 65%, respectively, of 37 patients undergoing vertebroplasty for malignant spinal lesions had sustained pain relief at 6 and 12 months postoperatively. Deramond and colleagues[19] suggested moderate to complete pain relief in 80% of 101 patients. Using kyphoplasty in 18 patients for treating vertebral compression fractures associated with multiple myeloma, Dudeney and colleagues[20] reported significantly improved quality of life through at least 52 months as measured using SF-36 scores. Pflugmacher and colleagues[21] reported significantly decreased pain and significantly improved function scores in a series of 20 patients through at least 12 months. Fourney and Gokaslan[14] reported that 84% of 56 patients, 21 with myeloma and 35 with primary spinal malignancy, had marked or complete pain relief through at least the first year.

Nevertheless, percutaneous vertebral body augmentation used for treating advanced spinal metastasis has not been widely adopted because it can be technically challenging to perform safely in this population. Most patients with metastatic lesions have epidural extension of the tumor, with possible disruption of the posterior cortical border. Complications associated with bone cement extravasation occur more often when treating patients with metastatic disease (up to 10%) than those with osteoporosis (1%–2%) or aggressive vertebral hemangiomas (2%–3%).[22] Mousavi and colleagues[23] reported that the risk of cement leakage during percutaneous vertebroplasty in the metastatic spine is significant, with up to 85.7% of procedures resulting in cement extravasation outside of the vertebral body. However, extravasation in these cases is not usually clinically significant. The higher risk of extravasation in patients with spinal malignancy, compared with patients with osteoporotic vertebra, may be attributed to the increased in situ pressures generated during the procedure.[24] Injection of bone cement into a vertebral body with a resident tumor is more difficult than into an osteoporotic vertebral body. The potential for eliciting tumor cell extravasation is a concern, and it deters many clinicians from using percutaneous vertebral body augmentation as a treatment option for patients with spinal metastasis.

Clearly, percutaneous vertebral body augmentation procedures can also be used in conjunction with conventional oncology therapies, including radiation therapy; however, the potentially significant clinical drawbacks have inhibited its use. Subsequently, clinical research in this area has tended to revolve around minimizing the limitations of using conventional vertebroplasty or kyphoplasty in this application by developing new techniques for permitting a safe and efficacious procedure.

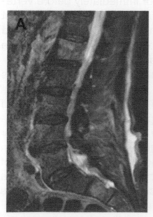 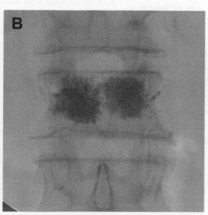 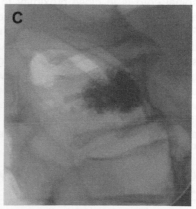

Fig. 2. A 78-year-old man with a history of lymphomatous involvement of L1 vertebral body. The disease involves the whole body of L1 with no epidural extension or paraspinal extension treated with standard vertebroplasty. (A) A sagittal T1-weighted image showing diffuse abnormal signals of L1 vertebra. (B, C) AP and lateral views, respectively, of postprocedure images.

ADAPTATIONS TO CONVENTIONAL VERTEBRAL BODY AUGMENTATION
Radiofrequency Ablation with Vertebroplasty

Grönemeyer and colleagues[25] were the first to report their clinical experience using radiofrequency ablation (RFA) of spinal tumors in combination with vertebroplasty. Patients had unresectable, osteolytic spine metastases and had not responded to radiotherapy or chemotherapy. The concept of using the combination of RFA and vertebroplasty caught on quickly as a technically innovative procedure for treating patients with metastatic spinal tumors. Immediately after Grönemeyer's report, several other investigators reported similar positive clinical outcomes in individual cases[26,27] and small case series[26,28] using this procedure.

A larger multicenter study (n = 43) was published in 2004.[29] All patients had tried and failed, or were ineligible for, receiving conventional treatments such as radiotherapy or surgery for treating spinal metastases. Before RFA treatment, patients had a mean pain score of 7.9 points; by 24 weeks posttreatment, the average pain score was reduced to 1.4 points. Complications observed with the procedure included second-degree skin burn at the grounding pad site (n = 1), transient bowel and bladder incontinence after the treatment of a metastasis involving the sacrum (n = 1), and fracture of the acetabulum after RFA of an acetabular lesion (n = 1). Longer-term follow-up of the same cohort was conducted to evaluate tumor progression and postoperative complications.[30] The mean time to tumor progression was 730 ± 54 days (Kaplan-Meier estimate).

When the posterior wall of the vertebra is compromised by the malignancy, RFA may pose a substantial risk for nerve damage because the spinal cord is in close proximity to the ablation field. Buy and colleagues[31] reported on a modified RFA delivery method that was designed to obviate the risk of inferring radiofrequency current into the spinal cord. Three patients with high-risk spinal tumors were treated. The RFA device that was used consisted of 2 needles (electrodes) that were activated in a bed of hypertonic saline (5.85%). This design allows more control over energy delivery than the conventional monopolar RFA technology.

Cryoablation with Vertebral Body Augmentation

If the lesion extends into the paravertebral area, a choice between standard RFA and cryoablation (CRA) can be used to control the soft tissue mass before the augmentation of the vertebral body. RFA requires heavy sedation or general anesthesia, which is not the case if CRA is used. Both techniques are usually performed under computed tomographic (CT) guidance[32] in a similar manner in other parts of the body. With CRA, an ice ball is created to ablate the soft tissue tumor. The size and location of such an ice ball can be accurately created under CT guidance, a benefit not available with RFA. After tumor ablation with RFA or CRA, the vertebral augmentation portion of the combined procedure is performed under direct visualization either by CT fluoroscopy, placing a C-arm in the CT suit, or by transferring the patient into the angiography room.

Tumor Debulking Combined with Vertebral Body Augmentation

In 2006, Tschirhart and colleagues[33] suggested tumor-volume reduction (as opposed to tumor necrosis occurring with RFA) be used in concert with vertebroplasty as a useful means for stabilizing vertebral bodies infiltrated by metastatic tumors. Using a biphasic parametric finite element analysis (FEA) model simulating a tumor infiltrated vertebral body at the lumbar level, the investigators reported that restoration of vertebral stability was theoretically possible after removing 30% of the tumor and inserting 1 to 2 mL of bone cement. The model indicated that creation of a cavity in the vertebra would permit preferential cement deposition in the region affected by lytic disease and facilitate restoration of stability because the region of lytic destruction and the surrounding bone would both be stabilized.

The following year, Ahn and colleagues[34] confirmed the use of Tschirhart's FEA model in cadaver tissues. Use of laser-induced thermotherapy to ablate the tumor immediately before vertebroplasty-facilitated bone cement placement improved biomechanical stability and reduced the risk of cement extravasation over using the vertebroplasty procedure alone.

Radiofrequency-based plasma ablation has become available as a method that can also be used to create a void in vertebral bodies affected by metastasis. This type of technology allows creation of a void in the tissue, similar to the laser devices, but is recognized to be safer to use in several clinical applications. With this type of device, radiofrequency energy is used to excite the electrolytes in a conductive medium, such as saline solution, creating precisely focused plasma. The energized particles in the plasma have sufficient energy to break molecular bonds, therefore having the ability to remove soft tissue at low temperatures, typically 40°C to 70°C. Georgy and

Wong[35] reported clinical feasibility and preliminary outcomes by using this type of device to make a void in the affected vertebral body before inserting bone cement. With this procedure, they found that it was possible to perform percutaneous cement augmentation in patients with advanced malignancy who would not normally be considered good candidates for undergoing conventional vertebroplasty or kyphoplasty. This technique was found to have the dual benefit of stabilizing the anterior column while minimizing the risk of anterior corpectomy by placing the injected cement in the anterior vertebral body, away from the compromised posterior wall (Fig. 3).[36]

It is important to point out that a cavity may be created using other methods such as balloon kyphoplasty. However, with balloon kyphoplasty,

the cavity is created by tissue displacement, and tumor tissue may encroach on the central canal. These issues do not occur with radiofrequency-based plasma ablation because a cavity intended for bone cement placement is created when tumor tissue is removed.

RECOMMENDATIONS FOR TREATMENT SELECTION

An algorithm for the percutaneous treatment of patients with spinal metastasis is presented in Fig. 4.

Before any percutaneous procedure in patients with spinal malignancy, both CT and magnetic resonance imaging (MRI) should be collected. The MRI allows assessment of the degree of compression, epidural extension, paraspinal extension,

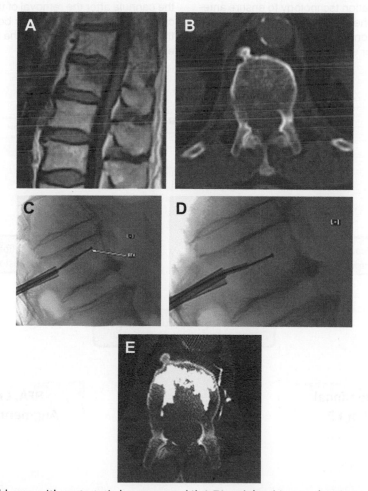

Fig. 3. A 78-year-old man with metastatic lung cancer. (A) A T1-weighted image showing a posteriorly located lesion. (B) An axial CT image confirming the finding in (A) and showing almost complete absence of the posterior cortical wall. (C, D) The Cavity SpineWand (ArthroCare Corp, Sunnyvale, CA, USA) creating a void in the anterior part of the vertebral body. (E) An axial CT image showing anterior deposition of the cement, with no leakage into the compromised posterior cortex.

presence of other lesions, and vascularity. The CT examination permits evaluation of bony architecture of the vertebral body and assessment of the posterior cortex and pedicles before augmentation, particularly in cases with cortical disruption and epidural extension.

As a general role, if the lesion is well confirmed inside the vertebral body with no cortical disruption or epidural extension, a standard vertebroplasty or kyphoplasty is performed. The author's preference is to perform standard vertebroplasty with highly viscous cement rather than kyphoplasty. The use of highly viscous cement is preferred to avoid any leakage. Because there are no indications for height restoration and because of risk of tumor tissue embolization by balloon inflation, kyphoplasty does not have real indications.

If there is cortical disruption or epidural extension (with no neurologic compromise), the author prefers using coblation technology to ensure anterior deposition of the injected cement. In presence of paraspinal lesions, treatment options include CRA or RFA with or without cement augmentation.

In such cases, the procedure is performed under CT guidance.

Bony landmarks may not be clear under fluoroscopy, particularly when the tumor extends into the pedicles. The tip of the needle should remain lateral to the medial border of the pedicle. If the pedicle cannot be seen, a posterolateral approach can be used. Alternatively, the location of the pedicle can be extrapolated by using the pedicles of the vertebral bodies above and below the affected level or by using neurologic monitoring techniques. If necessary, the entire procedure can be performed under CT guidance. If the posterior cortex is not intact, myelography can be performed immediately before injecting the bone cement so that any movement of the tumor mass into the thecal sac or neural foramen can be avoided during augmentation. Vascular tumors, such as renal cell carcinomas, may be associated with frank blood flow through the cannula after the removal of the stylet; the clinician must be prepared to lay bone cement along this track while withdrawing the needle to prevent excessive bleeding.

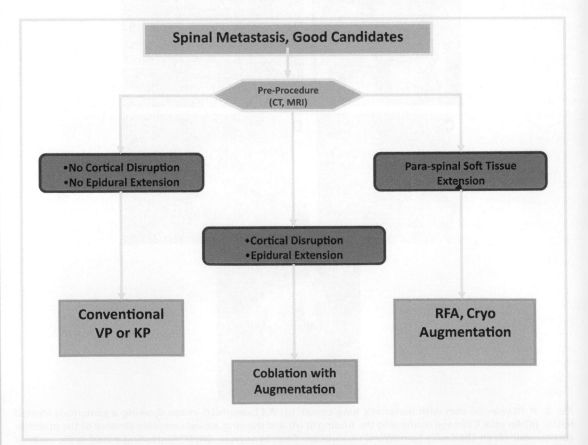

Fig. 4. A suggested algorithm for vertebral augmentation in different types of spinal lesions. (permission from AJNR). KP, kyphoplasty; MRI, magnetic resonance imaging; VP, vertebroplasty.

Placing bone cement into a vertebral body with a dense tumor mass is more difficult than placing cement into an osteoporotic vertebral body. Optimally, bone cement should be placed in the anterior aspect of the vertebral body so that maximum stability of the fractured vertebra can be achieved. Postprocedure examination using CT to evaluate the position of the cement, changes in the position of the tumor mass, cement leakage, iatrogenic fracture, or unsuspected hematoma is advocated.[10]

OPPORTUNITIES FOR FUTURE IMPROVEMENTS
Predicting Imminent Vertebral Body Compression Fracture

Learning to recognize patients who may be susceptible to a vertebral body compression fracture early in treatment may facilitate clinical outcomes. Hiroshi and colleagues[37] found that impending vertebral body collapse could be predicted using simple guidelines; they observed that compression fractures were most likely to occur under the following conditions:

1. 50% to 60% involvement of the vertebral body with no destruction of other structures
2. 35% to 40% involvement of vertebral body with 25% to 30% costovertebral joint destruction in the thoracic spine
3. 20% to 25% involvement of the vertebral body with destruction of posterior elements in the thoracolumbar and lumbar spine.

Routine evaluation using these criteria when providing care for patients with impending vertebral body collapse may improve patient outcomes rather than simply waiting for the vertebral body to fracture and then considering treatment.

Vertebral Body Augmentation with Hardware

Vertebral body augmentation has been described previously as beneficial for treating traumatic burst fractures where a short-segment pedicle screw fixation combined with vertebroplasty or kyphoplasty is used in lieu of traditional long-segment fusion.[38] Acosta and colleagues[39] concluded that kyphoplasty supplementation may improve the long-term integrity of short-segment pedicle screw constructs and allow for improved rates of fusion and better clinical outcomes in patients with traumatic lumbar burst fractures. Bone cement–augmented screw fixations have also been described previously.[40] Applications such as these could also potentially be developed for use in patients with bone malignancies, whereby

tumor debulking is performed before placing hardware and augmentation.

SUMMARY

Review of the current state of the art of percutaneous bone cement augmentation shows that this therapy provides a valuable addition to the current armamentarium for treating patients with vertebral body compression fractures associated with advanced spinal metastasis. Minimally invasive therapies are beneficial because complications and technical issues associated with open surgery are reduced and the number of patients ultimately receiving treatment earlier in the treatment algorithm will be increased.

REFERENCES

1. Krishnaney AA, Steinmetz MP, Benzel FC. Biomechanics of metastatic spine cancer. Neurosurg Clin N Am 2004;15:375–80.
2. Klimo P Jr, Schmidt MH. Surgical management of spinal metastases. Oncologist 2004;9:188–96.
3. Rios LAG, Melbert D, Krapcho M, et al, editors. SEER Cancer Statistics Review, 1975–2005. Bethesda (MD): National Cancer Institute. Available at: http://www.seer.cancer.gov/csr/1975_2005/. Based on November 2007 SEER data submission. Accessed August 7, 2007.
4. Adams N, Sonntag VK. Surgical treatment of metastatic cervical spine disease. Contemp Neurol 2001;23:1–5.
5. Dimar JR, Voor MJ, Zhang YM, et al. A human cadaver model for determination of pathologic fracture threshold resulting from tumorous destruction of the vertebral body. Spine 1998;23:1209–14.
6. Windhagen HJ, Hipp JA, Silva MJ, et al. Predicting failure of thoracic vertebrae with simulated and actual metastatic defects. Clin Orthop Relat Res 1997;344:313–9.
7. Denis F. The three column spine and its significance in the classification of acute thoracolumbar spinal injuries. Spine 1983;8:817–31.
8. Maranzano E, Latini P. Effectiveness of radiation therapy without surgery in metastatic spinal cord compression: final results from a prospective trial. Int J Radiat Oncol Biol Phys 1995;32:959–67.
9. Wu AS, Fourney DR. Evolution of treatment for metastatic spine disease. Neurosurg Clin N Am 2004;15: 401–11.
10. Jensen ME, Kallmes DE. Percutaneous vertebroplasty in the treatment of malignant spine disease. Cancer J 2002;8:194–206.

11. Matsubayashi T, Koga H, Nishiyama Y. The repara-tive process of metastatic bone lesions after radio-therapy. Jpn J Clin Oncol 1981;11:253.

12. Patel B, DeGroot H III. Evaluation of the risk of path-ologic fractures secondary to metastatic bone disease. Orthopedics 2001;24:612–7.

13. Regine WF, Tibbs PA, Young A, et al. Metastatic spinal cord compression; a randomized trial of direct decompression surgical resection plus radio-therapy vs. radiotherapy alone. Int J Radiat Oncol Biol Phys 2003;57:S125.

14. Fourney DR, Gokaslan ZL. Anterior approaches for thoracolumbar metastatic spine tumors. Neurosurg Clin N Am 2004;15:443–51.

15. Weinstein JN. Surgical approach to spine tumors. Orthopedics 1989;12:897–905.

16. Harrington KD. The use of methylmethacrylate for vertebral-body replacement and anterior stabiliza-tion of pathological fracture-dislocations of the spine due to metastatic malignant disease. J Bone Joint Surg Am 1981;63:36–46.

17. Cotten A, Dewatre F, Cortet B, et al. Percutaneous vertebroplasty for osteolytic metastases and myeloma: effects of the percentage of lesion filling and the leakage of methyl methacrylate at clinical follow-up. Radiology 1996;200:525–30.

18. Weill A, Chiras J, Simon JM, et al. Spinal metas-tases: indications for and results of percutaneous injection of acrylic surgical cement. Radiology 1996;199:241–7.

19. Deramond H, Depriester C, Galibert P, et al. Percu-taneous vertebroplasty with polymethylmethacry-late. Technique, indications, and results. Radiol Clin North Am 1998;36:533–46.

20. Dudeney S, Lieberman IH, Reinhardt MK, et al. Ky-phoplasty in the treatment of osteolytic vertebral compression fractures as a result of multiple myeloma. J Clin Oncol 2002;20:2382–7.

21. Pflugmacher R, Kandziora F, Schroeder RJ, et al. Percutaneous balloon kyphoplasty in the treatment of pathological vertebral body fracture and defor-mity in multiple myeloma: a one-year follow-up. Acta Radiol 2006;47:369–76.

22. Chiras J, Depriester C, Weill A, et al. [Percutaneous vertebral surgery. Technics and indications]. J Neu-roradiol 1997;24:45–59 [in French].

23. Mousavi P, Roth S, Finkelstein J, et al. Volu-metric quantification of cement leakage following percutaneous vertebroplasty in meta-static and osteoporotic vertebrae. J Neurosurg 2003;99:56–9.

24. Reidy D, Ahn H, Mousavi P, et al. A biomechan-ical analysis of intravertebral pressures during vertebroplasty of cadaveric spines with and without simulated metastases. Spine 2003;28: 1534–9.

25. Grönemeyer DH, Schirp S, Gevargez A. Image-guided radiofrequency ablation of spinal tumors: preliminary experience with an expandable array electrode. Cancer J 2002;8:33–9.

26. Masala S, Roselli M, Massari F, et al. Radiofrequency heat ablation and vertebroplasty in the treatment of neoplastic vertebral body fractures. Anticancer Res 2004;24:3129–33.

27. Schaefer O, Lohrmann C, Markmiller M, et al. Tech-nical innovation. Combined treatment of a spinal metastasis with radiofrequency heat ablation and vertebroplasty. AJR Am J Roentgenol 2003;180: 1075–7.

28. Van der LE, Kroft LJ, Dijkstra PD. Treatment of vertebral tumor with posterior wall defect using image-guided radiofrequency ablation combined with vertebroplasty: preliminary results in 12 patients. J Vasc Interv Radiol 2007;18:741–7.

29. Goetz MP, Callstrom MR, Charboneau JW, et al. Percutaneous image-guided radiofrequency abla-tion of painful metastases involving bone: a multi-center study. J Clin Oncol 2004;22:300–6.

30. Gevargez A, Groenemeyer DH. Image-guided radiofrequency ablation (RFA) of spinal tumors. Eur J Radiol 2008;65:246–52.

31. Buy X, Basile A, Bierry G, et al. Saline-infused bipolar radiofrequency ablation of high-risk spinal and paraspinal neoplasms. AJR Am J Roentgenol 2006;186:S322–6.

32. Moser T, Buy X, Goyault G, et al. Image-guided ablation of bone tumors: review of current tech-niques. J Radiol 2008;89:461–71.

33. Tschirhart CE, Finkelstein JA, Whyne CM. Optimization of tumor volume reduction and cement augmentation in percutaneous vertebroplasty for prophylactic treat-ment of spinal metastases. J Spinal Disord Tech 2006;19:584–90.

34. Ahn H, Mousavi P, Chin L, et al. The effect of pre-vertebroplasty tumor ablation using laser-induced thermotherapy on biomechanical stability and cement fill in the metastatic spine. Eur Spine J 2007;16(8):1171–8.

35. Georgy BA, Wong W. Plasma-mediated radiofre-quency ablation assisted percutaneous cement injection for treating advanced malignant vertebral compression fractures. AJNR Am J Neuroradiol 2007;28:700–5.

36. Georgy BA. Bone cement deposition patterns with plasma-mediated radiofrequency ablation and cement augmentation for advanced metastatic spine lesions. AJNR Am J Neuroradiol 2009;30: 1197–202.

37. Hiroshi T, Kiyoshi K, Naoki T, et al. Risk factors and probability of vertebral body collapse in metastases of the thoracic and lumber spine. Spine 1997;22: 239–45.

38. Cho DY, Lee WY, Sheu PC. Treatment of thoracolumbar burst fractures with polymethyl methacrylate vertebroplasty and short-segment pedicle screw fixation. Neurosurgery 2003;53:1354–60.

39. Acosta FL Jr, Aryan HE, Taylor WR, et al. Kyphoplasty-augmented short-segment pedicle screw fixation of traumatic lumbar burst fractures: initial clinical experience and literature review. Neurosurg Focus 2005;18:e9.

40. Jang JS, Lee SH, Rhee CH, et al. Polymethylmethacrylate-augmented screw fixation for stabilization in metastatic spinal tumors. Technical note. J Neurosurg 2002;96:131–4.

Sacral Fractures and Sacroplasty

Charles H. Cho, MD, MBA[a],*, John M. Mathis, MD, MSc[b],
Orlando Ortiz, MD, MBA[c,d]

KEYWORDS

- Sacral fracture • Sacroplasty • Treatment
- Bone augmentation

SACRAL FRACTURES

Incidence

Spontaneous, pathologic fractures of the sacrum are now well known, but were only first described as recently as 1982 by Lourie.[1] Such injuries are often termed as "insufficiency fractures," indicating that the bone strength is insufficient to withstand normal mechanical and physiologic forces.[2] The incidence of sacral insufficiency fractures (SIFs) is substantially less than that of osteoporotic fractures involving the lumbar and thoracic spine; however, in a published series evaluating elderly patients with acute onset of low-back pain and negative radiographs, bone scintigraphy diagnosed 102 sacral fractures over a 2-year period at a single institution.[3] In a second study,[4] using retrospective review of 1017 consecutive bone scans in patients older than 70 years, SIFs were identified in 194 patients (19%). Weber and colleagues[5] reported an incidence of 1.8% of SIFs (n = 20, total = 1015) in a female population, older than 55 years, admitted to a single department with low-back pain. In an active, single practice setting[6] that treated approximately 2000 patients with osteoporotic vertebral fractures, 80 patients with sacral insufficiency fractures were identified and treated, which was a relative incidence of at least 4%.

Reported data for incidence of localized sacral fractures from tumor destruction are limited at this time.

Causes of Sacral Fractures

Sacral fatigue or stress fractures occasionally occur in long-distance runners.[7] Sacral pathologic (insufficiency or tumor related) fractures may occur in patients with fragile or abnormal bone owing to osteoporosis, disorders of calcium metabolism, osseous metastatic disease, and prior radiation therapy.[2,5] Postmenopausal women with osteoporosis have been reported to be the most common group to suffer from sacral insufficiency fractures.[8]

Diagnosis

Sacral fractures present clinically with pain. Pain localizes mainly to the sacral and buttock region, but may be referred to the low lumbar spine.[8] Pain is usually acute in onset and exacerbated by weight bearing, which is typically relieved by rest or the supine position.[9] Referred pain to the hips or groin is common. For osteoporotic fractures, there can be concurrent fractures of the ischial and pubic rami,[5,10–12] or coexistent vertebral compression fractures.[5] There is usually no related neurologic abnormality.[8] Physical examination may show sacral tenderness on lateral

Disclosures: No disclosure, no industry affiliation or industry grants (C.H.C.). Industry/Government connections: Consultant, FDA-Orthopedics and Rehab Division (Washington, DC), Orthovita (Malvern, PA), Biomimetics (Nashville, TN), Crosstrees Medical (Denver, CO) (J.M.M.), Medtronic Spine (Memphis, TN) speakers bureau, SpineWave Inc (Shelton, CT) consultant (A.O.O.).
[a] Department of Radiology, Brigham and Women's Hospital, and Harvard Medical School, 75 Francis Street, Boston, MA 02115, USA
[b] Centers for Advanced Imaging, Roanoke, VA 24014, USA
[c] Department of Radiology, Winthrop-University Hospital, 259 First Street, Minneola, NY 11501, USA
[d] Stony Brook University School of Medicine, Stony Brook, NY 11794, USA
* Corresponding author.
E-mail address: ccho81@partners.org

compression,[8] and there is restricted mobility that is indistinguishable from sacroiliac arthropathy and other spinal and pelvic pathologic conditions.

Conventional plain radiographs are insensitive, only occasionally showing sclerosis of the sacrum or an actual fracture line.[8] Computed tomography (CT) offers greater sensitivity (Fig. 1); however, acute, nondisplaced fractures without sclerosis may be difficult to visualize.[13] Bone scintigraphy is reliable, but with less anatomic detail compared with CT. Bone scintigraphy demonstrates increased tracer activity in the areas of the fracture (Fig. 2).[8] Ambiguity on bone scan in this region is common because of bowel and bladder activity or uptake around the sacroiliac (SI) joint caused by degenerative change. Careful attention to findings on the posterior nuclear images is therefore helpful when evaluating the sacral region.

Magnetic resonance (MR) imaging is sensitive and specific in demonstrating sacral fractures.[14] Marrow edema is visible as decreased signal on the T1-weighted images. T2-weighted short tau inversion recovery (STIR) or fat-saturated T2-weighted images show increased signal related to edema (Fig. 3). Axial or coronal images show the fractures in 2 complementary planes. Although sacral insufficiency fractures demonstrate enhancement after intravenous contrast agent administration, this often is not required because the imaging findings on the unenhanced MR imaging examination are fairly characteristic. In a patient with tumor history, sacral fractures may be misinterpreted as metastatic disease,[9] which sometimes can be differentiated with diffusion-weighted images.[15]

Sacral Fracture Types

The classic appearance of a sacral insufficiency fracture on skeletal scintigraphy is an H-shaped uptake pattern (Fig. 4). This pattern results from fractures of the sacral ala bilaterally with a horizontal fracture component that extends through the central sacrum (usually at about the S2 level).[1] The fracture may present with only the vertical component on one or both sides of the sacrum. The horizontal fracture may also accompany a single unilateral component. The complexity of the fracture makes the diagnosis difficult based solely on the bone scan, thus anatomic confirmation with CT or MR imaging is always preferred.

Functional Outcome of Sacral Fractures

Functional outcome data are limited for sacral insufficiency fractures with few reported series. In a series of 60 hospitalized patients (mean age of 83 years) with pelvic insufficiency fractures, of which 16 involved the sacrum, the average hospital stay was 45 days. After 1 year, only 36.6% had the same level of self-sufficiency as before the fracture and 25% were discharged to institutions with a 1-year mortality of 14.3%.[16] Less bleak outcomes have also been reported. In a series of 20 patients with sacral insufficiency fractures (mean age of 74 years), 17 patients had resolution of local pain and 3 patients required analgesics for pain control.[8] In another series of 20 hospitalized patients with sacral insufficiency fractures (mean age 79), with analgesics and physical therapy, pain resolved for all 20 patients at 9 weeks.[5] In patients with sacral fractures associated with tumor, functional outcomes data are more limited because these are patients with shorter life expectancy directly related to the tumor.

TREATMENT OPTIONS

Medically, patients with insufficiency fractures are treated with medications to reverse osteoporosis and to decrease pain.[17] Early mobilization is recommended[5,17,18] to stimulate osteoblastic bone-forming activity by weight bearing or muscle tension strength. Prolonged immobilization leads to bone resorption, complications of sacral decubitus ulcers, and deep venous thromboses.[17]

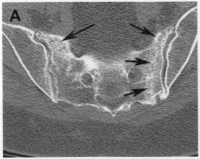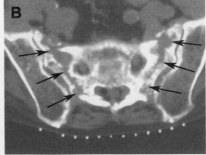

Fig. 1. (A) Computed tomography (CT) scan. The sacral fracture is indicated by the arrows. In this figure it is detectable but less obvious than in B. Some fractures may present with only minor discontinuities at the bone margins. (B) CT scan. Arrows indicate the bilateral alar fractures of the sacrum. These fractures are much more obvious than in A.

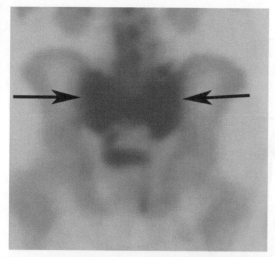

Fig. 2. Bone scintigraphy of pelvis, posterior view. Abnormal activity in the sacrum caused by a sacral insufficiency fracture. The arrows point to the abnormal uptake in the lateral margins of the sacrum.

Rehabilitation therapy is recommended.[16,17] Surgery is usually not considered for insufficiency fractures because most patients are treated conservatively,[9] as surgery is rarely indicated.[17]

However, surgery remains available with attempts to bridge the fractured ala areas with metallic screws placed via a lateral approach through the SI joints.

For pain and fractures from invasion of tumor, surgery is extensive, with high morbidity and complications.[19–21] Patients with metastatic lesions who continue to have pain after radiotherapy and chemotherapy are considered for surgery. However, surgical fusion with hardware would be extensive, involving the lumbar spine to bilateral ileum,[22] and postoperative complication rates for spine surgery from metastatic disease are high.[21]

Percutaneous sacroplasty is an image-guided percutaneous injection of bone cement into the sacral fracture site. The proposed mechanism of pain relief is fracture stabilization that eliminates motion of the fractured bone. Although the concept of vertebroplasty (injection of cement into compressed thoracic and lumbar vertebral bodies) theoretically applies to sacral fractures as well, even experienced practitioners were initially hesitant to apply vertebroplasty techniques at the sacral level. This hesitance was, in part, due to constraints imposed by the complex sacral

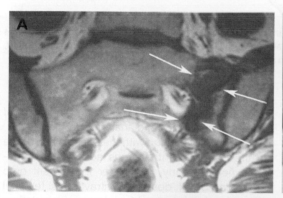

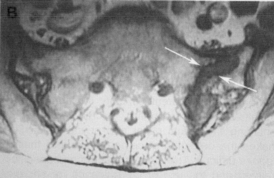

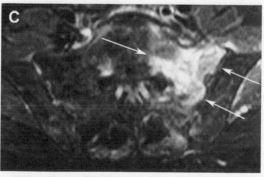

Fig. 3. (A) Coronal T1 magnetic resonance (MR) image. Arrows point to the unilateral sacral fracture. The fracture line is dark on T1 imaging. (B) Axial T1 MR image. Arrows indicate the unilateral sacral fracture. (C) Inversion recovery MR image. Arrows point to the sacral fracture. The actual fracture line is less distinct compared with A and B. However, the marrow signal abnormality associated with the edema is much more obvious with the fat suppression.

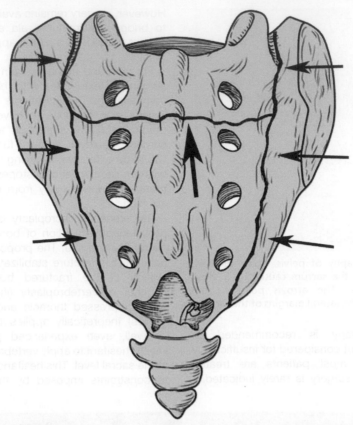

Fig. 4. The usual location of the fracture lines in the sacrum with a typical H-shaped pattern. Lateral fracture lines usually extend between the sacroiliac joints and the neural foramina. These lines can extend into the foramina or, rarely, the spinal canal. The central component usually traverses the transmembrane segment S2 region.

anatomy. The inherent difficulty in fluoroscopic visualization of important sacral landmarks, including the spinal canal and neural foramina, makes the detection of cement leaks into these spaces difficult. The authors recommend specific training and the use of CT guidance for sacroplasty.[22–24] In a prospective, multicenter, observational study of 52 patients treated with sacroplasty, there was a statistically significant immediate improvement with dramatic decrease in pain after the procedure.[25]

SACROPLASTY TECHNIQUE

Appropriate patient selection is critical to ensure a favorable outcome. Sacroplasty should be offered to patients with severe pain, poorly responsive to conventional medical therapy. Patients unable to tolerate strong pain medications or patients with tumor involvement with continued pain after radiation, chemotherapy, or both are also potential candidates for sacroplasty. Fractures should be documented by scintigraphy, CT and/or MR imaging.

The authors prefer MR imaging for its combination of sensitivity, specificity, and anatomic detail.

Sacroplasty is begun with the patient lying prone on the CT table. Intravenous sedation is sometimes needed early to transfer the patient onto the table. Small doses of intravenous fentanyl and midazolam are used for intravenous sedation, titrated to the patient's pain. Monitoring of vital signs and oxygen saturation levels are routine.

Intravenous antibiotics are recommended and given at the start of the procedure. Cephazolin, 1 g intravenously, is commonly used. If the patient is allergic to cephalosporin or penicillin, an alternative is 1 dose of clindamycin, 600 mg, plus ciprofloxacin, 400 mg intravenously.

After a lateral CT scout image, 3-mm axial images through the sacrum are obtained with a skin grid. Puncture sites are localized and marked on the skin. Sterile preparation of the target area with surgical drapes is used. Surgical hand-washing techniques with cap, mask, and sterile gown and gloves are used as per sterile protocol.

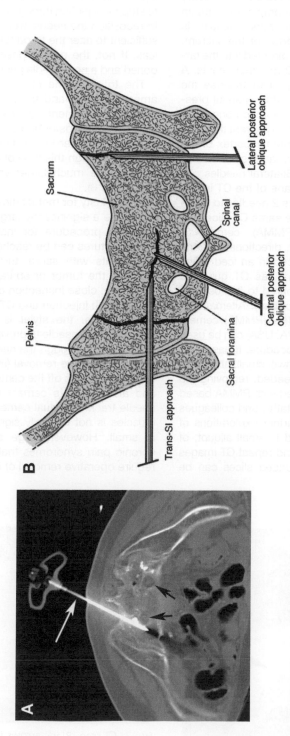

Fig. 5. (A) CT scan. The white arrow points to the bone biopsy needle placed into the sacral fracture, avoiding the sacral foramina (black arrows) and sacral iliac joint. (B) The potential needle introduction trajectories. A trans-sacroiliac approach is possible, but injection of cement should avoid the joint even if the route passes through it.

Local anesthetic with lidocaine, 1% or 2%, is used to infiltrate the subcutaneous tissue and the periosteum of the sacrum at the intended needle entry site. Through a small dermatotomy made with an 11-gauge scalpel blade, a bone needle is advanced to the posterior cortex of the sacrum. With CT images, the needle is directed into the targeted fracture line in 5- to 10-mm increments. A sterilized mallet may be helpful to traverse the cortex or areas of sclerotic matrix; manual pressure is sufficient through osteoporotic bone.

Extreme care must be taken to prevent the bone needle from traversing the anterior cortex of the sacrum; the neural foramina and spinal canal should be avoided (**Fig. 5**). Bilateral needles can be placed in a single scan plane of the CT image (**Fig. 6**). This positioning allows 2 needles to be injected and monitored with the same CT slice.

Polymethylmethacrylate (PMMA) cement is mixed per the manufacturer directions and the delivery syringes can be placed in an iced saline bath to increase working time, as CT guidance requires additional time compared to fluoroscopic guided percutaneous vertebroplasty. Alternatively, the recently FDA approved (non-PMMA) cement Cortoss (Orthovita; Malvern, PA, USA) can be used to great advantage in this procedure. It has a mix on demand system that allows small aliquot of cement to be mixed when needed, removing the time constraints normally faced with PMMA based cements. See the article by Mathis and colleagues elsewhere in this issue for further explorations of this topic. Cement is injected in small aliquot, of approximately 0.3 to 0.5 ml and repeat CT images are obtained (3–5 closely spaced slices can be

focused on the needle tips and do not need to cover the entire sacrum). The cement fill is meticulously monitored and any evidence of leak is an indication to stop the injection through that needle. An attempt to reposition the needle within the fracture may be sufficient to alter the fill pattern and prevent further leak. If not, the needle position should be abandoned and a new needle position obtained.

The total volume of cement used is variable among patients and fractures. Usually, the total amount of cement ranges from 5 to 15 mL (**Fig. 7**). Some osteoporotic areas in the sacrum actually form large cavities. When a fracture extends through this type of lesion, reinforcement may require much larger volumes for adequate filling (**Fig. 8**).

Sacroplasty for metastatic infiltration is believed to require a significantly larger volume of cement than the procedure for insufficiency fracture.[22] Most fractures can be reached with CT guidance. In patients with sacral tumor, the cement will displace the tumor or spread around the tumor. Therefore, close inspection of the sacral foramina during each injection and CT imaging is needed.

If possible, the stylet is inserted before the removal of the needle to prevent tracking of cement in the needle through the needle path. Rotation of the needle before removal (even without replacing the stylet) breaks off the cement at the needlepoint and also prevents cement deposition along the needle track. Residual cement in the paraspinous muscles is not clinically significant if the quantity is small. However, large amounts can create chronic pain syndromes that may be severe and require operative removal of cement.

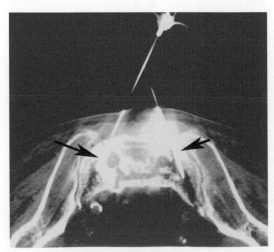

Fig. 6. Axial CT scan. Placement of bilateral needles (*arrows*) through sacral fractures.

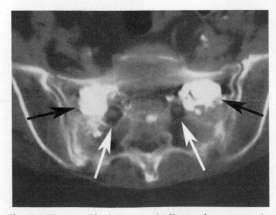

Fig. 7. CT scan. Black arrows indicate the cement injected into the bilateral alar fractures. White arrows point to the neural foramina. Actual cement volumes are empiric and must be determined at the time of treatment to adequately cover the fracture territory.

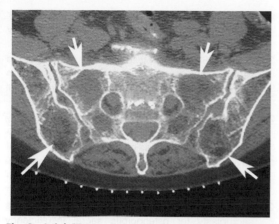

Fig. 8. Axial CT scan. Arrows point to the areas devoid of trabeculae in this osteoporotic individual. The voids create cavities within the bone that requires larger than usual volumes of cement to adequately fill.

After satisfactory placement of the cement, needles are removed and sterile dressing is placed over the puncture site. The patient is carefully rolled to the bed and is on bed rest, with no axial loading for 1 to 2 hours. After 2 hours of uneventful recovery, the patient can ambulate and be discharged.

Fluoroscopy has been used for sacroplasty, but because of the limited anatomic resolution, CT is preferred and recommended.[23] For patients with tumor burden in the sacrum with substantial sacral destruction, CT is thought to be the optimum imaging method.[22] There is mixed opinion about CT fluoroscopy. Quick images can be obtained with CT fluoroscopy, although evaluation in the cranial-caudal dimension may be difficult.[24,26] In patients with a large body size, resolution is limited and CT fluoroscopy may not be helpful.

CODING AND REIMBURSEMENT

Previously, a specific code for sacroplasty was not available; thus an unlisted code (22899) and supervision and interpretation code (72292) CT guidance was used. Starting in 2010, a category III temporary code is available for percutaneous sacral augmentation (sacroplasty) for uniteral (0200T) or bilateral injections (0201T). For radiological supervision and interpretation, 72291 and 72292, and if bone biopsy is performed 20220 and 20225 are available.[27] The procedure report should document the need for the surgery, including the appropriateness and description of the procedure.

SUMMARY

Sacral pathologic fractures from insufficiency and tumor-related causes can create severe pain in affected patients. For insufficiency fractures, sacroplasty is recommended for patients with severe pain who cannot tolerate medications, or with other medical comorbidities that may predispose the patient to further complications from bed rest or rehabilitation. For patients with continued pain from tumor involvement after radiation or chemotherapy, sacroplasty is recommended as a palliative treatment option.

REFERENCES

1. Lourie H. Spontaneous osteoporotic fracture of the sacrum. An unrecognized syndrome of the elderly. JAMA 1982;248:715–7.
2. Pentecost RL, Murray RA, Brindley HH. Fatigue, insufficiency, and pathologic fractures. JAMA 1964; 187:1001–4.
3. Hatzl-Griesenhofer M, Pichler R, Huber H, et al. The insufficiency fracture of the sacrum. An often unrecognized cause of low back pain: results of bone scanning in a major hospital. Nuklearmedizin 2001; 40(6):221–7.
4. Wat SY, Seshadri N, Markose G, et al. Clinical and scintigraphic evaluation of insufficiency fractures in the elderly. Nucl Med Commun 2007;28(3): 179–85.
5. Weber M, Hasler P, Gerber G. Insufficiency fractures of the sacrum. Spine 1993;18(16):2507–12.
6. Cho C, Kortman K, Mathis J. Sacroplasty. In: Mathis JM, Golovac S, editors. Image guided spine intervention. 2nd edition. New York: Springer; 2010. p. 355–74.
7. Major NM, Helms CA. Sacral stress fractures in long-distance runners. AJR Am J Roentgenol 2000;174: 727–9.
8. Gotis-Graham I, McGuigan L, Diamond T, et al. Sacral insufficiency fractures in the elderly. J Bone Joint Surg Br 1994;76:882–6.
9. Tsiridis E, Upadhyay N, Giannoudis PV. Sacral insufficiency fractures: current concepts of management. Osteoporos Int 2006;17:1716–25.
10. Aretxabala I, Fraiz E, Perez-Ruiz F, et al. Sacral insufficiency fractures. High association with pubic rami fractures. Clin Rheumatol 2000;19: 399–401.
11. Davies AM, Evans NS, Struthers GR. Parasymphaseal and associated insufficiency fractures of the pelvis and sacrum. Br J Radiol 1988;61(722):103–8.
12. Peh WC, Khong PL, Ho WY, et al. Sacral insufficiency fractures. Spectrum of radiological features. Clin Imaging 1995;19(2):92–101.
13. Grangier D, Garcia J, Howarth NR, et al. Role of MRI in the diagnosis of insufficiency fractures of the sacrum and acetabular roof. Skeletal Radiol 1997; 26(9):517–24.

14. Brahme SK, Cervilla V, Vint V, et al. Magnetic resonance appearance of sacral insufficiency fractures. Skeletal Radiol 1990;19:489–93.

15. Byun WM, Jang HW, Kim SW, et al. Diffusion-weighted magnetic resonance imaging of sacral insufficiency fractures. Spine 2007;32(26):E820–4.

16. Tailandeler J, Langue F, Alemanni M, et al. Mortality and functional outcomes of pelvic insufficiency fractures in older patients. Joint Bone Spine 2003;70: 287–9.

17. Lin JT, Lane JM. Sacral stress fractures. J Womens Health (Larchmt) 2003;12:879–88.

18. Babayev M, Lachmann E, Nagler W. The controversy surrounding sacral insufficiency fractures: to ambulate or not to ambulate? Am J Phys Med Rehabil 2000;79(4):404–9.

19. Akasu T, Yamaguchi T, Fujimoto Y, et al. Abdominal sacral resection for posterior pelvic recurrence of rectal carcinoma: analyses of prognostic factors and recurrence patterns. Ann Surg Oncol 2007; 14(1):74–83.

20. Matsuo T, Sugita T, Sato K, et al. Clinical outcomes of 54 pelvic osteosarcomas registered by Japanese musculoskeletal oncology group. Oncology 2005; 68:375–81.

21. Pascal-Moussellard H, Broc G, Pointillart V, et al. Complications of vertebral metastasis surgery. Eur Spine J 1998;7:438–44.

22. Wee B, Shimal A, Stirling AJ, et al. CT-guided sacroplasty in advanced sacral destruction secondary to tumour infiltration. Clin Radiol 2008;63:906–12.

23. Zhang J, Wu C, Gu Y, et al. Percutaneous sacroplasty for sacral metastatic tumors under fluoroscopic guidance only. Korean J Radiol 2008;9:572–6.

24. Layton KF, Thielen KR, Wald JT. Percutaneous sacroplasty using CT fluoroscopy. AJNR Am J Neuroradiol 2006;27:356–8.

25. Frey ME, DePalma MJ, Cifu DX, et al. Percutaneous sacroplasty for osteoporotic sacral insufficiency fractures: a prospective, multicenter, observational pilot study. Spine J 2008;8:367–73.

26. Butler CL, Given CA 2nd, Michel SJ, et al. Percutaneous sacroplasty for the treatment of sacral insufficiency fractures. AJR Am J Roentgenol 2005;184: 1956–9.

27. Lawler GJ. Spinal injection procedures: update on billing and coding. In: American Society of Spine Radiology Annual Symposium: Las Vagas, NV, February 18–21, 2010. p. 586.

Percutaneous Therapy for Symptomatic Synovial Cysts

John M. Mathis, MD, MSc[a],*, Orlando Ortiz, MD, MBA[b,c]

KEYWORDS
- Synovial cyst • Synovial cyst rupture • Spine pain
- Epidural cyst

Synovial cysts are extradural lesions that appear to arise from the synovial lining of the facet joints.[1–4] The cause and mechanism of development are thought to be micromotion and microtrauma that are associated with degenerative changes within the facet joint. This condition leads to the rupture of synovial membrane and subsequent cyst formation caused by the leak of synovial fluid and cells. There is containment of this material with proliferation of mesenchymal cells and myxoid degeneration.[5] The most common location of cysts is the L4-L5 level because it is the location reported to have the highest degree of spinal motion (**Fig. 1**).[6,7] These cysts are almost always associated with significant degenerative facet disease and, not uncommonly, a degree of degenerative spondylolisthesis is also present.

When they are small, synovial cysts are usually asymptomatic. However, there may be symptoms of back pain related to degenerative facet disease. As the cysts enlarge, they can compress the thecal sac or the exiting nerve root in the foramina. This compression may result in spinal stenosis and/or radiculopathy (**Fig. 2**). Symptoms are usually unilateral but, with progressive spinal stenosis, bilateral symptoms can also occur. Bilateral cysts are rarely present (see **Fig. 2**). Synovial cysts are unusual in higher locations (cervical and thoracic) but can produce myelopathy when present.

The differential diagnoses of cyst-like lesions in this location include arachnoid cysts, perineural (Tarlov) cysts, schwannomas, disk fragments, ganglion cysts, cysts of the ligamentum flavum or posterior longitudinal ligament, and pseudocysts.[8,9] The most common cyst in the L4-L5 area is the synovial cyst. Arachnoid cysts are more common in the thoracic region. Tarlov cysts and schwannomas have direct association with the nerve root and are generally found away from the facet joint. Schwannomas enhance uniformly, whereas a synovial cyst will show rim enhancement only. Most cysts will be high signal on T2 and low signal on T1 magnetic resonance (MR) images (see **Figs. 1** and **2**). Atypical signal patterns occur because calcification in the rim (and sometimes center) of the cysts is not uncommon (**Fig. 3**). In addition, air can occasionally be found inside these cysts and comes from the degenerative facet joint.

Synovial cysts are conspicuous on MR imaging, and this method is currently the most common method of diagnosis.[1,8,10] Computed tomography (CT) can also be used for diagnosis[11,12] but is less common now. Increased awareness of this lesion

Disclosures: Industry/Government connections: Consultant, FDA-Orthopedics and Rehab Division (Washington, DC), Orthovita (Malvern, PA), Biomimetics (Nashville, TN), Crosstrees Medical (Denver, CO) (J.M.M.). Speakers Bureau, Medtronic Spine (Memphis, TN), Consultant, SpineWave Inc (Shelton, CT) (O.O.).
a Centers for Advanced Imaging, Roanoke, VA 24014, USA
b Department of Radiology, Winthrop-University Hospital, 259 First Street, Mineola, NY 11501, USA
c Stony Brook University School of Medicine, Stony Brook, NY, USA
* Corresponding author.
E-mail address: jmathis@rev.net

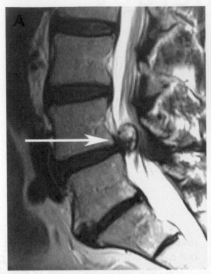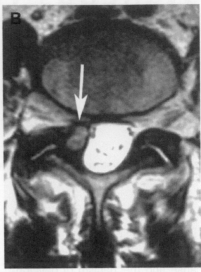

Fig. 1. (*A*) Sagittal T2-weighted magnetic resonance (MR) image. The arrow points to a synovial cyst at the L4-L5 level. The cyst is high signal on this sequence. (*B*) Axial T2-weighted MR image. The arrow again points out the synovial cyst. There is lateral pressure on the thecal sac and the exiting nerve. The high signal part of the cyst represents only a portion of the cyst components that create local mass effect.

and its conspicuous nature on an MR image make it a progressively more common diagnosis.

TREATMENT OPTIONS

Traditional therapy has been surgical microdecompression and removal of the symptomatic synovial

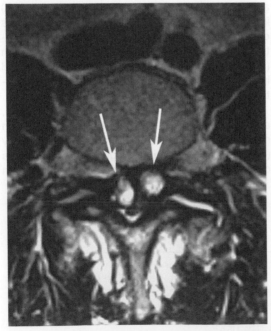

Fig. 2. Axial T2-weighted MR image. The 2 arrows point to bilateral synovial cysts. These cysts completely compress the thecal sac at this level and create severe spinal stenosis.

cyst. Surgery by removal of the compression on the adjacent structure works well for pain relief. However, surgery alone does not address the facet degeneration or spondylolisthesis (if present). If spondylolisthesis is present, surgical fusion to address the slip may be indicated. In the Mayo Clinic[6] experience (involving 194 patients), 91% of the patients had good pain relief, and 84% experienced improvement in motor deficits. However, complications included 4 patients subsequently requiring fusion because of spondylolisthesis that developed after laminectomy, cerebrospinal fluid leak (in 3 patients), discitis (1 patient), epidural hematoma (1 patient), seroma (1 patient), deep vein thrombosis (1 patient), and a death caused by cardiac arrhythmia.

Percutaneous facet or cyst injection (without cyst distension or rupture) has been reportedly successful in some patients, but the recurrence of symptoms is high.[13,14] In a long-term follow-up, it was seen that the condition of approximately only one-third of the patients improved. Most patients had poor outcomes, and more than half of them went on to undergo surgery.

Percutaneous injection of the synovial cyst with attempts at rupture or overdistension has also been reported in various articles.[10,15,16] In each of these articles, there is improved outcome compared with using an injection alone. Two studies respectively report 75%[10] and 72%[15] long-term good outcomes with injection. Some patients had recurrence of pain and went on to have a second attempt at cyst rupture. The least encouraging study reported that approximately

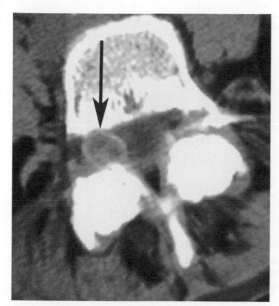

Fig. 3. Axial CT image. The arrow points to a synovial cyst with calcified rim. Note the hypertrophy around the facet joints caused by degenerative change.

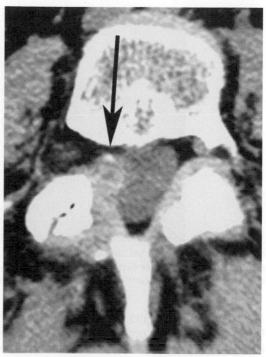

Fig. 4. Axial CT image. The arrow points to the synovial cyst. The cyst can be differentiated from the facet joint and thecal sac without contrast injection.

50% of patients in their series had long-term benefits.[16] This number is an improvement when compared with using an injection alone, with these patients avoiding surgery. The patients treated with injection and cyst rupture and who improved had long-term outcomes similar to patients who had surgery. As reported in the Mayo Clinic experience,[6] surgery was not without notable complication. This risk seems to be averted in the percutaneous group making a first attempt at cyst rupture a reasonable, less invasive choice.

PERCUTANEOUS TECHNIQUE

This procedure is performed with the patient in the prone position. The patient's skin is prepared with a sterile solution. Because the procedure is often transiently painful (during cyst distension), conscious sedation is commonly used. This sedation is preceded by a preoperative workup and perioperative monitoring. Preoperative antibiotics may also be administered; usually, 1 g of Ancef is given intravenously.

Image guidance for this procedure can be obtained with either fluoroscopy or CT. Fluoroscopy gives real-time visualization of needle placement but is problematic because the cyst can usually not be visualized directly. However, contrast injection into the facet joint (that the cyst communicates with) usually opacifies the cyst. One can then directly stick the needle into the cyst (via an interlaminar approach) or attempt distension and

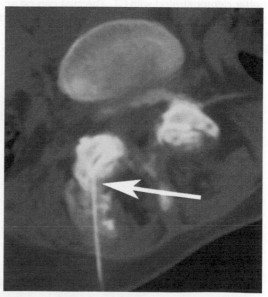

Fig. 5. Axial CT image. The arrow points to the needle-entry point into the degenerated facet joint. Direct puncture of the facet joint can be difficult because of the proliferative changes that can block access.

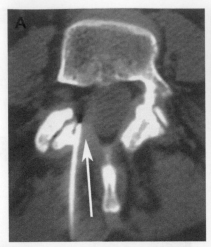
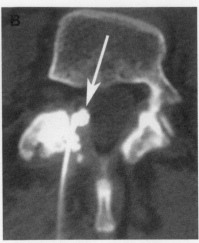

Fig. 6. Axial CT image. (*A*) The arrow shows the access to the synovial cyst via an intralaminar approach. This approach allows the needlepoint to penetrate the cyst directly. (*B*) The arrow points to contrast in the synovial cyst that is injected to confirm appropriate needle location.

rupture by injecting into the facet joint directly. Direct puncture of the cyst seems to have a greater likelihood of creating enough pressure to rupture the cyst, but both techniques have been successful.

CT guidance, like fluoroscopy, has its advantages and disadvantages. Contrast resolution is better with CT, frequently allowing the cyst to be seen before direct injection (Fig. 4). Needle placement into the facet joint is also facilitated because the 3-dimensional contour of the facet joint is better demonstrated with CT. The cyst can be accessed via injection into the facet joint itself (Fig. 5). Direct puncture of the cyst via an interlaminar approach can also be accomplished with CT (Figs. 6 and 7), but the gantry angle required to allow this approach may be problematic. This latter problem has been minimized with the use of CT fluoroscopy.

A 20- or 22-gauge spinal needle is used. Smaller needles will substantially restrict the rate of fluid injection and may make overdistension of the cyst difficult. Small syringes (3-, 5-, or 10-mL) are used.

Regardless of the imaging technique used, access to the facet joint or direct puncture of the cyst allows the operator to attempt overdistension of the cyst to produce cyst rupture. Injection of radiographic contrast (that is approved for intrathecal use) should precede cyst rupture (Fig. 8).

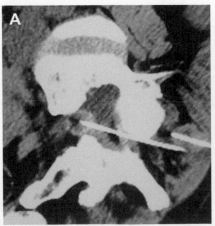
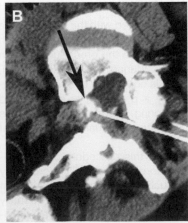

Fig. 7. Axial CT image. (*A*) This image shows intralaminar access to the synovial cyst from the opposite side. This patient had a scoliotic spine with considerable proliferative change around facet joints. This route resulted in the best access (access via the ipsilateral foramina was blocked by bowel). (*B*) The arrow points to contrast injected into the synovial cyst to confirm accurate needle placement.

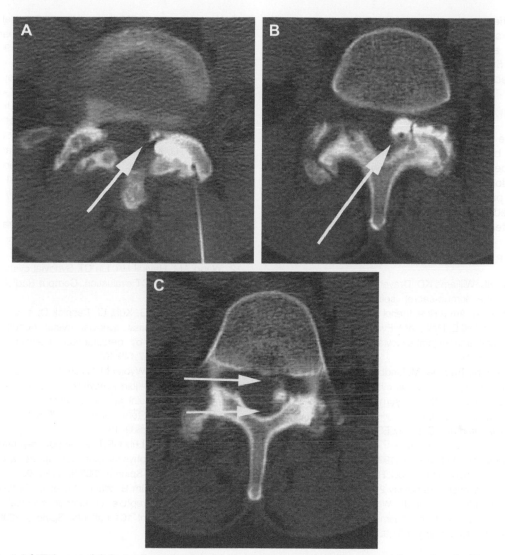

Fig. 8. Axial CT image. (*A*) A needle in the facet joint allows contrast filling of the joint and early filling of the communicating synovial cyst (*arrow*). (*B*) Progressive injection of contrast shows the synovial cyst (*arrow*) filled to capacity. (*C*) The synovial cyst after rupture contains only a small amount of residual contrast. Ill-defined contrast from the rupture is seen in the adjacent epidural space (*arrows*).

This injection is useful to prove communication with the cyst through the facet joint or determine the appropriate needle position when direct puncture is used.

A total volume of 4 to 5 mL of injectate is used to produce overdistension of the cyst. The injection rate should be sufficiently brisk so that cyst rupture is likely. The injectate should contain a corticosteroid (equivalent to 80 mg of Depo-Medrol, Pharmacia & Upjohn, Bridgewater, NJ, USA). In addition, 1 to 3 mL of a local anesthetic is included (such as 0.25% bupivacaine). The final volume is adjusted as needed with normal saline. With the rupture of the cyst, the injectate is dispersed into the epidural space, and serves to reduce pain locally and to add a persistent anti-inflammatory effect that aids recovery (see **Fig.** 8C).

Postoperative imaging is usually more definitive with CT than with fluoroscopy. If rupture is accomplished, the procedure is terminated, and the patient will be transferred to an appropriate holding area for monitoring. If the recovery is uneventful, the patient can be discharged within 1 to 2 hours after the procedure. The patient should initially be ambulated with assistance because the effect of a successful cyst rupture is somewhat equivalent to a nerve root block. The patient may have transient leg weakness on the side of the cyst rupture.

Patients who have recurrent symptoms with a persistent cyst visualized on imaging should have a second attempt at cyst rupture. More than 50% of these patients will be successfully treated with a second procedure.

SUMMARY

Image-guided synovial cyst puncture and rupture have been shown to be effective in a significant number of individuals, allowing pain relief and functional recovery without surgery. This outpatient procedure is safe and easily tolerated. The procedure should be discussed with patients as an alternative to surgery.

REFERENCES

1. Liu SS, Williams KD, Drayer BP, et al. Synovial cysts of the lumbo-sacral spine: diagnosis by MR imaging. Am J Roentgenol 1990;154:163–6.
2. Apostolaki E, Davis AM, Evans N, et al. MR imaging of lumbar facet joint synovial cysts. Eur Radiol 2000; 10:615–23.
3. Tillich M, Trummer M, Lindbichler F, et al. Symptomatic intraspinal synovial cysts of the lumbar spine: correlation of MR and surgical findings. Neuroradiology 2001;43:1070–5.
4. Howington JU, Connolly ES, Voorhies RM. Intraspinal synovial cysts: 10 year experience at the Ochsner Clinic. J Neurosurg 1999;91(2):193–9.
5. Marichal DA, Bertozzi JC, Rechtine G. Lumbar facet synovial cysts. Radiology 2006;241(2):618–21.
6. Lyons MK, Atkinson JL, Wharen RE, et al. Surgical evaluation and management of lumbar synovial cysts. J Neurosurg 2001;93(1):53–7.
7. Yarde WL, Arnold PM, Kepes JJ, et al. Synovial cysts of the lumbar spine: diagnosis, surgical management, and pathogenesis. Surg Neurol 1995;43: 459–65.
8. Jackson DE, Atlas S, Mani JR. Intraspinal synovial cysts: MR imaging. Radiology 1989;170:527–30.
9. Christophis P, Asamoto S, Kuchelmeister K. Juxtafacet cysts, a misleading name for cystic formations of mobile spine. Eur Spine J 2007;16(9):1499–505.
10. Bureau NJ, Kaplan PA, Dussault RG. Lumbar facet joint synovial cyst: percutaneous treatment with steroid injection and distention-clinical and imaging follow up in 12 patients. Radiology 2001; 221:179–85.
11. Hemminghytt S, Daniels DL, Williams AL. Intraspinal synovial cysts: natural history and diagnosis by CT. Radiology 1982;145:375–6.
12. Wang AM, Haykal HA, Lin CT. Synovial cysts of the lumbar spine: CT evaluation. Comput Radiol 1987; 11:253–7, 170.
13. Bjorkengrem AG, Kurz LT, Resnick D, et al. Symptomatic intraspinal synovial cysts: opacificationi and treatment by percutaneous injection. Am J Roentgenol 1987;149:105–7.
14. Parlier-Cau C, Wybier M, Nizard R, et al. Symptomatic lumbar facet joint synovial cysts: clinical assessment of facet joint steroid injection after 1 and 6 month and long-term follow-up in 30 patients. Radiology 1999;210:509–13.
15. Allen TL, Tatli Y, Lutz GE. Fluoroscopic percutaneous lumbar zygapophyseal joint cyst rupture: a clinical outcome study. Spine J 2009;9(5):387–95.
16. Martha JF, Swaim B, Wang DA, et al. Outcome of percutaneous rupture of lumbar synovial cysts: a case series of 101 patients. Spine J 2009;9(8): 572–6.

Epidural Steroid Injections

John M. Mathis, MD, MSc

KEYWORDS

- Pain management • Epidural steroid injection
- Spine pain • Conservative pain management
- Nerve block • Nerve root block

Low-back and neck pain are frequent complaints among patients, as well as a leading cause of doctor visits and loss of work in the United States each year. It is estimated that up to 5% of adults seek medical attention for back pain annually.[1] The cost of back pain exceeds 100 billion dollars in the United States alone.[2] Many of these patients may proceed to surgery in an attempt to eliminate pain and recover functionality, which adds additional cost and complexity to the treatment paradigm and is now believed to offer no long-term advantage compared with more conservative treatment modalities for the vast majority of patients experiencing pain without motor symptoms.[3] In the prospective Spine Patient Outcomes Research Trial (SPORT), surgery was found effective for rapid pain relief but both groups (surgical and conservative management) faired similarly in matched-control comparisons at 2-year follow-up. There was no demonstrated risk in undergoing conservative management compared with early surgical intervention (a long-term warning that has been heard from surgeons lobbying against conservative treatment and for early surgery).

Because many patients will recover from back pain without surgery, it seems reasonable, as well as cost effective, to try conservative therapy in the vast majority of patients before progressing to surgery. Epidural steroid injections (ESIs) serve as a part of a conservative, therapeutic approach to pain management in these individuals.

HISTORY

Epidural injections of anesthetics were reported over a century ago in Europe.[4] Steroid injections into the epidural space began in the 1950s.[5] Since then, there have been numerous publications attempting to analyze the results of these injection procedures for control of back and radicular pain.[6–12] The results are mixed, and most opinions can be supported by selected data. Therefore, trying to prove utility, or not, is difficult on the basis of available data (much of which was anecdotal and without control). There is definitely a body of information that indicates improved outcome (reduced pain and quicker return to work) with epidural steroids.[11,13] Those who administer ESIs daily in pain practices see a substantial percentage of patients who get welcome benefit from these simple procedures. They have become a common component in the process of providing pain relief and increased mobility while patients undergo other rehabilitation procedures and recovery.

Historically, referrals for ESIs came from surgeons. Patients were sent to them by primary care providers for surgical evaluation. Many patients had been treated with pain medicines and had been waiting for the magic referral only to find out that now they would need to have imaging, rehabilitation, or ESI. It is likely that the process had already been weeks long. Today, ESI referrals are more often directly from the

Disclosures: Industry/Government connections: Consultant, Food and Drug Administration-Orthopedics and Rehabilitation Division (Washington, DC), Orthovita (Malvern, PA), Biomimetics (Nashville, TN), Crosstrees Medical (Denver, CO).
Centers for Advanced Imaging, Roanoke, VA 24014, USA
E-mail address: jmathis@rev.net

Neuroimag Clin N Am 20 (2010) 193–202
doi:10.1016/j.nic.2010.02.006

primary care physician. The process of ESI can be started early while the patient is waiting to see the surgeon. This allows early intervention of pain and better participation in the rehabilitation procedures while awaiting the surgical consult (which could be canceled as pain improves with conservative treatment and time).

PATIENT SELECTION

The patient considered for an ESI experiences pain that originates from the area to be treated. Patients with a short history of pain seem to do better than those with chronic pain (for longer than 6 months).[8] Patients with pain resulting from disc herniation respond better to ESI than do patients with pain resulting from spinal stenosis.[9] Patients who have not been operated on get better relief than those previously operated on and with epidural scar. Prior operation, chronic pain, or pain resulting from spinal stenosis is not a contraindication but does suggest that there will likely be a poorer outcome than for other groups.

Imaging is always helpful to correlate anatomic defects or abnormalities with the clinical presentation. However, imaging does not visualize pain, and, therefore, the clinical examination is of primary importance in determining where treatment should be applied. If there are no specific contraindications to ESI, the ESI can be initiated on the basis of clinical findings before imaging or while waiting for imaging to be obtained.

CONTRAINDICATIONS

Because ESI is an injection into a space that contains vascular elements and that is out of reach to direct pressure, it cannot be used in patients who are on anticoagulants or who have coagulation defects. Coumadin and heparin obviously are contraindications to ESI because of the risk of epidural hematoma. Even with the use of 25- or 27-gauge needles, the risk is not completely eliminated. Less clear is the risk for patients taking platelet inhibitors such as aspirin or ticlopidine. Guidelines for cessation of antiplatelet drugs before epidural injections vary; so each individual society should be checked for their most recent recommendations. The American Society of Regional Anesthesia recommends being off ticlopidine for 14 days and off clopidogrel for 7 days. Recommendations are less specific for aspirin but seem to vary between 5 to 7 days.[14]

Diabetes is not a contraindication, but steroid injections raise glucose levels and make their control more erratic for several days. Patients with brittle diabetes or those with poor control may need medication changes or closer monitoring after ESI.

ESI for patients with active infection (during antibiotic therapy) should usually be postponed until therapy is completed and signs of infection have cleared.

IMAGE GUIDANCE

ESI without image guidance should be avoided. Evaluations have shown a 25% to 40% miss rate when these injections are performed without guidance.[15,16] Misplaced injections result in lesser pain relief and raise the risk of secondary complications from steroid placed in unwanted locations such as the intrathecal space. Intrathecal steroid injections are associated with arachnoiditis.

Generally, fluoroscopy is the method of choice for ESI. It offers quick, accurate, and cost-effective image guidance. Johnson and colleagues[17] used fluoroscopy-guided ESIs in a large cohort of more than 5000 patients, with a complication rate of 0.07%. Several reports have described computed tomography (CT) for guidance, but all have comprised small numbers of patients and were anecdotal in quality. There is no proof that CT offers any advantage over fluoroscopy for safety and is definitely negative for time efficiency and cost.

TECHNICAL CONSIDERATIONS

Local anesthesia is used before the introduction of the epidural needle. One percent lidocaine with bicarbonate is a commonly used local anesthetic. This material still has considerable sting and discomfort. For this reason, the author prefers a "no sting" mix that includes lidocaine, bicarbonate, and Ringer lactate (Table 1). This mixture eliminates essentially all the discomfort to the anesthetic. It contains no preservative, and any excess must be discarded at the end of each day.

The needles used for ESI by the anesthesiologist were traditionally of the Tuohy type. This needle was rather blunt (to protect from easy puncture of the dura) and large (14 to 18 gauge). With image guidance there is no need for needles of this size or type. Routine use of a 25- or 27-gauge spinal (Quinke) needle allows easy epidural access with minimal trauma and discomfort.

Epidural injection of radiographic contrast is commonly done with image guidance to confirm appropriate epidural positioning before steroid injection. Nonionic contrast approved for intrathecal use is recommended, which prevents complications with inadvertent intradural injections. In patients with contrast allergy, loss of

Table 1
"No sting" anesthetic solution

Solution	Lidocaine (4%) (mL)	Lactated Ringer (mL)	Bicarbonate (mL)	Epinephrine
1	4	24	2	0 mL
2	4	24	2	0.15 mL (1:1000)

Solution 1 makes a sting-free local anesthetic with 0.5% lidocaine. Solution 2 is similar to solution 1 but contains 1:200,000 epinephrine. Both solutions should be mixed on the day of use and discarded daily as they contain no preservatives. The total volume of each solution is 30 mL.

resistance technique can be used with only minimal loss of accuracy, as image guidance is still used for regional needle localization. This technique does eliminate the opportunity to prevent intravascular needle placement (and negative aspiration for blood does not exclude the possibility of intravascular positioning).[18]

Some operators perform a full epidurogram before injecting steroids,[17] although not necessary in the routine procedure. The epidurogram adds volume to the procedure (which can be problematic as some patients experience local pain during injection), and the information gained is rarely used to change the procedure in any meaningful way. Only a small volume of contrast, usually no more than 1 to 2 mL, is needed to confirm appropriate epidural location before injecting steroid. A small volume is all that is needed to insure that an intravascular position has been avoided as well. The site of the injection should be the expected site of abnormality based on clinical presentation. In some patients with spinal stenosis, injection of the level above is necessary to prevent barotrauma that can be produced by adding fluid volume to an already tight space. By injecting above the level, gravity helps move the steroid solution into the adjacent level while avoiding the barotrauma. Transforaminal injection in this situation is also a consideration.

ESI is usually a minimally painful procedure. Patients often experience a feeling of pressure but actual pain is uncommon. Pain may result from injecting too rapidly and discomfort can be volume related. When there is pain or discomfort, simply stopping or slowing the injection often results in quick subsidence or reduction of the discomfort. The injection can be completed with a slower infusion rate. Pain that is persistent or not responsive to stopping the injection should be a sign to move the injection to an adjacent level or to use another administration route. Paresthesia or pain can be a sign of an intraneural injection.

Transforaminal injections are an alternative to the traditional interlaminar route. Although low in risk (in the hands of an experienced operator), this route should be used for specific indications and not as the initial or routine method. There is more pain and discomfort associated with the transforaminal route and also more chance of complication. Complications with this method are rare in the lumbar area but frequent enough in the cervical region that some pain practices have abandoned this method entirely. The use of CT, nonparticulate steroid (dexamethasone), or needle placement within a specific location within the foramina does not eliminate this risk. The operator is faced with a potentially devastating complication (cervical cord or brainstem stroke) while trying to treat a benign disease with a temporary therapy. This is a sure prescription for a lost malpractice case. (The author stopped doing cervical transforaminal injections in 2005 because of the awareness of multiple such malpractice cases and has seen no significant loss of effectiveness with standard cervical ESI alone.)

After a successful injection, the patient is returned to the observation area or waiting room and released after a 30-minute interval of uneventful recovery.

There is a long history of use associated with ESI treatments that have contributed to an entrenched dogma concerning the number of injections per year and interval between injections. None of these beliefs are based on scientific data or significant trial outcomes and therefore should be flexible. Treatment should be individualized to the patient's presentation, needs, and response to therapy. The author routinely sees ESI patients for a reevaluation in 7 to 14 days after the prior treatment. Based on response to therapy, a repeat ESI is performed as needed at that time. Only 3 ESIs in a 6-month period, fewer if possible, are recommended to limit steroid exposure. The usual limit of 3 injections is more a historical one than a hard limit and can be adjusted as needed for some individuals. (However, if 3 or 4 injections do not fix the problem, then neither will 30.)

ANATOMIC REGION
Lumbar and Sacral

The lumbar region is the most commonly treated area, and the usual ESI approach is via an interlaminar route (transforaminal and caudal routes are alternatives but used less frequently). The level and side of the abnormality are determined by imaging and clinical means. The patient is placed prone on the radiographic table and sterile skin preparation applied to the area to be treated. The exact site is determined with fluoroscope imaging, and the site marked for the placement of local anesthetic. A 25- or 27-gauge spinal (Quinke) needle is then introduced and advanced toward the chosen spinal interlaminar location with fluoroscopic guidance (**Figs. 1** and **2**). Once the appropriate trajectory for the interlaminar approach is established (see **Fig. 2**A), the fluoroscope is moved from the posterior-to-anterior (PA) projection to a shallow oblique position, away from the side of needle entry (see **Fig. 2**B). This allows one to view the needle from a lateral projection and determine the depth of the needle tip as it is advanced. The needle is advanced through the interlaminar space and just beyond the posterior laminar line on the oblique projection. A small amount of contrast (or saline when using loss-of-resistance technique) is now injected, and a lentiform configuration of the contrast

should be seen within the epidural space (see **Fig. 2**C). The posterior margin of the contrast is contained by a straight or slightly curved line created by the posterior laminar ligaments. (If contrast does not pool or collect locally then one must assume an intrathecal or intravascular injection and steroid should not be administered at this location.) With the epidural space confirmed, the steroid injection can proceed (see the following pharmacology section for dosages by route and anatomic area).

The caudal and transforaminal routes are used for specific indications that include

1. Prior surgery in the lumbar area with obliteration or scarring of the epidural space
2. Spinal stenosis and pain produced during an interlaminar injection
3. Clinical or anatomic problems involving the low sacrum or coccyx area
4. Lack of response to standard interlaminar injections.

The caudal route is generally an easy anatomic approach for epidural injection but requires needle entry low in the perianal crease making it seem more invasive to the average patient. However, it provides useful access to the sacrum, coccyx, and the low lumbar epidural space. The coccygeal hiatus (**Fig. 3**A) can be palpated and then confirmed fluoroscopically. After sterile skin preparation, local anesthesia is applied and a 25-gauge spinal needle advanced into the hiatus. This is best guided by lateral fluoroscopy (**Fig. 3**B). A slight

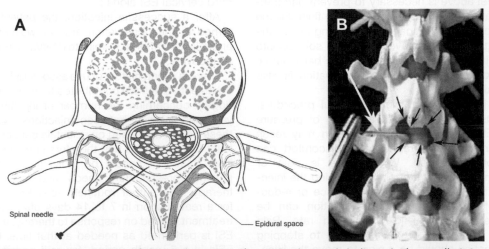

Fig. 1. (*A*) An axial cross section of the lumbar spine. The epidural space is indicated. The needle is introduced into the posterior epidural space via the traditional intralaminal approach. (*B*) Small black arrows outline the intralaminar space, which provides the usual window into the epidural space. The large white arrow points to the spinal needle entering the epidural space via this window through a slightly oblique approach.

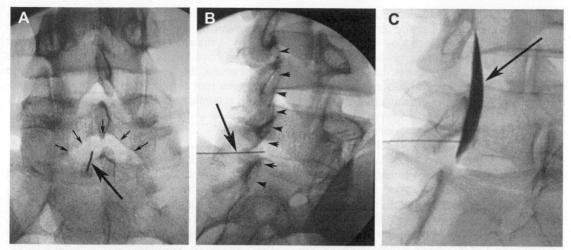

Fig. 2. (A) Anterior-posterior fluoroscopic image. The large black arrow points to the spinal needle approaching the epidural space via the intralaminar route. Small black arrows outline the margins of the intralaminar space. (B) Oblique fluoroscopic image (away from the side of the needle introduction). The large black arrow indicates the spinal needle. This projection allows one to accurately gauge the needle depth. The small arrows show the posterior spinal laminar line. This line is visualized in the oblique projection as the opposite posterior elements are superimposed. This line marks the superficial margin of the epidural space and indicates the minimal depth that the needle must be introduced. (C) Oblique fluoroscopic image. The black arrow points to radiographic contrast collecting in the epidural space (epidurogram), which is the typical lentiform shape seen in this location. Note the relatively straight margin on the needle side. This margin is formed by the posterior laminar ligaments.

curve is placed on the needle so that entry into the hiatus can be facilitated. The needle is advanced 1 to 2 cm into the caudal epidural space, and contrast injected to confirm an appropriate location. One should see good epidural spread of contrast without flow into the vascular or intradural space (Fig. 3C). The volume of injection used is larger in this area, as the steroid is pushed over a wider area compared with a standard lumbar ESI.

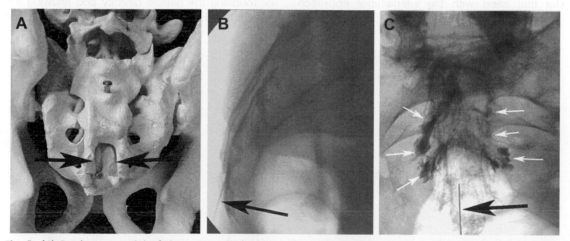

Fig. 3. (A) Sawbones model of the sacrum and coccyx. The 2 black arrows point to the coccygeal hiatus. This anatomic feature can be palpated directly to localize the area for needle entry. (B) Lateral fluoroscopic image of the sacrum and coccyx. The black arrow points to the spinal needle entering the coccygeal hiatus. Note the needle angle. It is parallel to the posterior bone margin, which allows the needle to extend through the hiatus and into the epidural space beyond. This angle is necessary to achieve movement of contrast into the epidural space. (C) Anterior-to-posterior fluoroscopic image. The large black arrow points to the spinal needle entering the epidural space via the caudal hiatus. Small white arrows indicate radiographic contrast spreading through the epidural space in the sacral region.

The intent of a transforaminal ESI is delivery of steroid into the epidural space for pain therapy. This is different from a selective nerve block, which deposits the injectate in the foramen and lateral to the ganglion. A selective nerve block is usually used as a diagnostic procedure to confirm a specific nerve source of pain (although steroid is also often included in the injection). The transforaminal route theoretically provides an alternate route to the epidural space with the entry point usually chosen to provide maximal steroid coverage for the suspected area of abnormality. Because access to the epidural space via this route requires deeper penetration into the foramen than is necessary with a nerve block (generally needle placement must be beyond or medial to the ganglion), this procedure is often more uncomfortable to the patient as the exiting nerve sheath is at risk of direct puncture.

The transforaminal approach begins with an oblique PA approach of the needle on the side to be treated. The needle (25- or 27-gauge spinal needle) is directed into the upper foramen beneath the margin of the pedicle of the level above (**Fig. 4**A). Once the trajectory is established, the fluoroscope is returned to a straight PA position. In this projection, the needle is advanced to the inside margin of the pedicle (**Fig. 4**B). Contrast is introduced to ensure that there is no intravascular or intrathecal penetration. With the fluoroscopy turned obliquely away from the side of injection (similar to the angle used for an interlaminar ESI), the contrast in the epidural space should look like that seen with the interlaminar approach (**Fig. 4**C). This is an ESI that simply uses a different route for epidural access. The contrast therefore is in the same space and will look just like that seen with the intralaminar approach. If the contrast does not have this distribution but stays outside the foramina, the injection is postganglionic and is a nerve root block. Once correct needle positioning is confirmed, the steroid is injected.

Cervical

The epidural space in the cervical region is smaller than that found in the lumbar area. The most common site for interlaminar access is C5-C6. As with the lumbar injection, the procedure is started with the patient in the prone position. Sterile skin preparation and local anesthesia are used as before. With fluoroscopy in the anterior-to-posterior projection, the interlaminar location is visualized (**Fig. 5**A) and a 25- or 27-gauge spinal needle introduced and appropriate trajectory established. The fluoroscope is moved to the lateral projection to visualize the depth of the needle for its final advancement. As the needle passes the posterior laminar line, contrast is injected to demonstrate the epidural space (**Fig. 5**B). Spread of contrast is similar to the lumbar area, but because of the small size of the space, only a fraction of a milliliter may be seen to cover several anatomic levels (**Fig. 5**C, D). It is important to use a small connecting tubing on the needle (with internal volume, or dead space, of <0.5 mL), which allows the contrast syringe to be exchanged for the steroid syringe without moving or touching the needle directly and allowing the needle tip to stay within the small epidural space

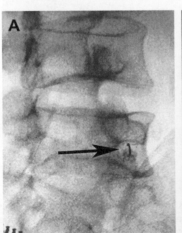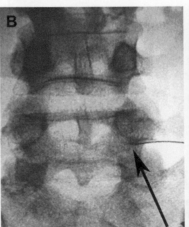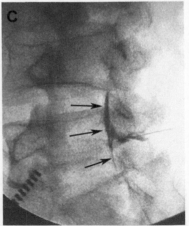

Fig. 4. (*A*) Oblique fluoroscopic image. The black arrow points to the spinal needle introduced just below the margin of the pedicle (into the upper portion of the selected neural foramina). (*B*) anterior-to-posterior fluoroscopic image. In this projection, the needle is advanced until the tip is along the inner margin of the pedicle (*black arrow*). (*C*) Oblique fluoroscopic image. The black arrows show the typical spread of contrast in the epidural space.

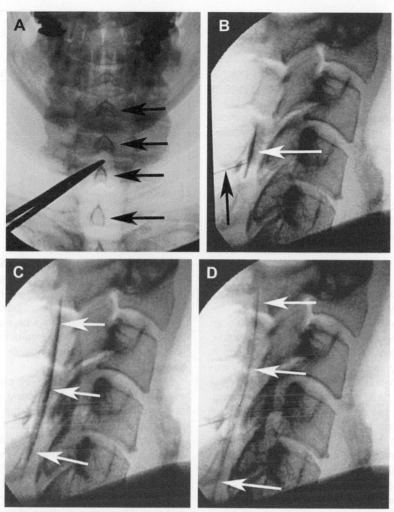

Fig. 5. (*A*) Anterior-to-posterior fluoroscopic image. In this projection, the posterior cervical spinous processes are indicated by the black arrows. This image allows easy identification of the cervical level to be injected. (*B*) Lateral fluoroscopic image. The black arrow points to the spinal needle, which is introduced to just beyond the posterior spinal laminar line. Injection of contrast reveals a typical epidural spread (*white arrow*). (*C*) Lateral fluoroscopic image. White arrows point to epidural spread of contrast. Less than 0.5 mL of contrast shows posterior distribution over 3 cervical levels. (*D*) Lateral fluoroscopic image. White arrows point to the epidural contrast. The spread is wider than in (*C*) and is less dense. This spread is produced as the steroid solution is injected into spinal needle and washes out the less-than-1 mL of contrast used. A total volume of 3 mL of is injected, and good multilevel coverage is achieved.

reliably during syringe exchange. The small volume or dead space of the tube reduces the amount of contrast that has to be injected ahead of the steroid mixture. The total volume injected into the cervical area is small (usually 3 mL) compared with the lumbar area, but still wide coverage can be expected. Slow injection is advised as this region is sensitive to volume changes and local pain can be created quickly. Indeed, patients who are prone to migraine headaches may experience headache symptoms after a cervical epidural injection. In this case, treatment for the headache should be the usual therapy that the patient relies upon.

As stated previously, the author has discontinued cervical transforaminal (nerve root) injections because of the potential for permanent neurologic complications related to it. No reduction in outcome response has been noted over the 4 years that this change has been in place.

PHARMACOLOGY

The materials used for epidural injections are discussed in more detail, see the article by Mathis and colleagues elsewhere in this issue for further exploration of this topic.

ESIs (all anatomic regions) use similar doses of steroid, although the total volume injected may vary. Caudal injections use a volume of approximately 15 mL; lumbar, 7 to 10 mL; and cervical, 3 mL. Volumes are achieved by adding normal saline to the steroid and anesthetic dosages selected.

No anesthetic is added to the cervical injection. Rarely, anesthetic in this region has been implicated in difficulty with breathing. Therefore, only steroid and normal saline are used in the cervical region.

The dosage of steroid will depend on the steroid type (**Table 2**). The common methylprednisolone (Depo-Medrol) dosage is 80 mg. An equivalent of triamcinolone (Kenalog) or betamethasone (Celestone) can be substituted (**Table 3**). Short-acting steroids, such as dexamethasone, have been used but seem to have a less-prolonged effect at pain relief.

Anesthetic use in the injection is more a historic finding than a necessity. As the anesthetic dosage is increased, there is an increasing chance of anesthetic nerve blockade. In the lumbar area this nerve blockade results in lower extremity numbness and motor dysfunction, which can last several hours and, if unexpected by the patient, may be very distressing. In the cervical region, breathing dysfunction or apnea may result. As this procedure should be essentially pain free, anesthetic is not required and indeed adds nothing to the long-term outcome. However, if a patient is in extreme pain before the procedure, anesthetic in small amounts can be helpful in the short term. Bupivacaine (0.25%) can be added in the caudal and lumbar regions in doses of 1 to 3 mL with little consequence.

COMPLICATIONS

In the hands of experienced operators, complications are rare in any of these procedures. Most problems are minor and self-limiting. Headache may be the most common complication of ESI and can result from several causes. Steroids can

Table 3
Approximate equivalent glucocorticoid dosages

Drug	Equivalent Dose (mg)
Cortisone	30
Hydrocortisone	25
Prednisone	6
Prednisolone	6
Methylprednisolone	5
Triamcinolone	5
Dexamethasone	1
Betamethasone	1

produce headache in some individuals, who require only symptomatic therapy. Spinal headache, resulting from inadvertent puncture of the thecal sac, may require blood patch.

Epidural or subarachnoid bleeding is rare and prevented by judicious avoidance of patients who are on anticoagulants or on antiplatelet therapy.

Direct vascular injection of steroid is usually avoided by real-time monitoring of the injection of contrast before injection of the steroid. (This is possible with fluoroscopy but not CT.) Aspiration is a poor substitute for direct visualization for detecting whether the needle is intravascular in location. Neither technique is reliable 100% of the time. The risk of stroke following steroid injection is also much less in the lumbar region compared with the cervical. Although a plethora of vessels exist in the neural foramina in the cervical and lumbar regions, these do not usually feed directly into the cord in the lumbar area (**Fig. 6**). (Rarely a long recurrent radicular branch will feed from the low lumbar or sacral region back to the area of the conus.)

In the cervical region, stroke may be caused by 2 mechanisms. One is injection of a particulate steroid into a feeding artery, which can usually be protected against by direct visualization of a contrast injection preceding the steroid. The second mechanism is direct injury to the vessel by the needle. Radicular arteries in the cervical region are only about 150 μm in size and can be transected or dissected by a spinal needle. This injury may not result in stroke if sufficient collateralization exits (a common occurrence in the cervical cord). However, as is always the case, there is no guarantee and some areas of the cord will be at risk of stroke with this injury.

In the cervical area, most foramina have radicular branches that directly supply the anterior or posterior surface of the cord. These are always at risk

Table 2
Recommended dosages of typical steroid preparations used in ESIs

Steroid	Dose (mg)
Depo-Medrol	40–80
Kenalog	40–80
Celestone	6–12
Dexamethasone	6–12

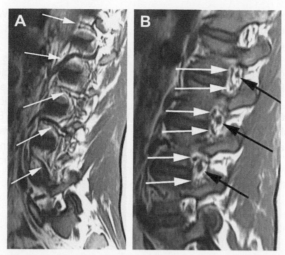

Fig. 6. (*A*) Sagittal magnetic resonance (MR) image of the spine. A sagittal image along the lateral margin of the lumbar spine shows the multiple vessels (venous and arterial) that traverse the margin of the vertebral bodies on their way to supply the neural foramina (*white arrows*). The lumbar region is chosen for demonstration because of its larger size compared with the cervical zone. Vessels are actually more numerous in the cervical region. (*B*) Sagittal MR image of the spine. White arrows point to the multiple vessels that penetrate the neural foramina to supply nerve, bone, and joint structures. Black arrows indicate lumbar nerves. The vascular location and number of vessels vary from foramina to foramina in all anatomic areas.

with cervical intraforaminal injections because there is no fixed location of these vessels and specific placement of the needle within the foramina does not guarantee vascular avoidance. If one stays sufficiently outside the foramina to avoid the vessels, the injection effectively becomes a nerve root block and not a transforaminal epidural.

SUMMARY

ESIs have become a common part of conservative therapy for spine and radicular pain. As this form of pain is often self-limited, all forms of conservative therapy should be used before surgery when the problems do not include motor dysfunction. ESI is very safe if judiciously applied and it should be available as part of every image-guided interventional practice.

REFERENCES

1. Rubin DI. Epidemiology and risk factors for spine pain. Neurol Clin 2007;25:353–71.
2. Katz JN. Lumbar disc disorders and low-back pain: socioeconomic factors and consequences. J Bone Joint Surg Am 2006;88(Suppl 2):21–4.
3. Weinstein JN, Tosteson TD, Lurie JD, et al. Surgical versus nonoperative treatment for lumbar disk herniation: the Spine Patient Outcomes Research Trial (SPORT): a randomized trial. JAMA 2006;296:2441–50.
4. Sicard MA. Les injections medicamenteuses extradurales par voie sacro-coccygienne. C R Soc Dev Biol 1901;53:396–8.
5. Robecchi A, Capra R. Hydrocortisone, first clinical experiments in the field of rheumatology. Minerva Med 1952;43:1259–63.
6. Berman AT, Garbarino JL Jr, Fisher SM, et al. The effects of epidural steroid injection of local anesthetics and cortocosteroids on patients with lumbosacral pain. Clin Orthop 1984;188:144.
7. Bowman SJ, Wedderburn L, Whaley A, et al. Outcome assessment after epidural corticosteroid injection for low back pain and sciatica. Spine 1993;18:1345.
8. Heyse-Moore GH. A rational approach to the use of epidural medication in the treatment of sciatic pain. Acta Orthop Scand 1978;29:366.
9. Rivest C, Katz JN, Ferrante FM, et al. Effects of epidural steroid injection on pain due to lumbar spinal stenosis or herniated disks: a prospective study. Arthritis Care Res 1998;11:291.
10. Landau WM, Nelson DA, Armon C, et al. Assessment: use of eipidural steroid injections to treat radicular lumbosacral pain: report of the Therapeutics and Technology Assessment Subcommittee of the American Academy of Neurology. Neurology 2007;69:614.
11. Bush K, Hillier S. A controlled study of caudal epidural injections of triamcinolone plus procaine for the management of intractable sciatica. Spine 1991;16:572–5.
12. Carette S, Leclaire R, Marcoux S, et al. Epidural corticosteroid injections for sciatica due to herniated nucleus pulposus. N Engl J Med 1997;336:1634–40.

13. Dilke TF, Burry HC, Grahame R. Extradural cortico-steroid injection in management of lumbar nerve root compression. Br Med J 1973;2:635.

14. Horlocker TT, Wedel DJ, Benzon H, et al. Regional anesthesia and the anticoagulated patient: defining the risks (the second ASRA Consensus Conference on Neuraxial Anesthesia and Anticoagulation). Reg Anesth Pain Med 2003;28:172–97.

15. White AH. Injection techniques for the diagnosis and treatment of low back pain. Orthop Clin North Am 1983;14:553–67.

16. White AH, Derby R, Wynne G. Epidural injections for the diagnosis and treatment of low-back pain. Spine 1980;5:78–86.

17. Johnson BA, Schellhas KP, Pollei SR. Epidurography and therapeutic epidural injections: technical considerations and experience in 5334 cases. AJNR Am J Neuroradiol 1999;20:697–705.

18. Renfrew DL, Moore TE, Kathol MH, et al. Correct placement of epidural steroid injections: fluoro-scopic guidance and contrast administration. AJNR Am J Neuroradiol 1991;12:1003.

Radiofrequency Neurolysis

Stanley Golovac, MD

KEYWORDS

- Radiofrequency • Low back pain • Lumbosacral facet joint
- Lumbar anatomy • Lumbar joint injections

Lumbar facet joints were recognized as potential sources of back pain by Goldthwait as early as 1911.[1] The term facet syndrome, defining lumbosacral pain with or without sciatic pain, was coined by Ghormley in 1933.[2] Badgley[3] in 1941 suggested that facet joints themselves could be a primary source of pain separate from spinal nerve compression pain; he attempted to explain the role of facet joint pain in large numbers of patients with low back pain whose symptoms were not caused by a ruptured disc. Multiple investigators[3–9] described the pattern of pain caused by facet joint stimulation. Bogduk and colleagues[10] showed that facet joint pain can be relieved by anesthetizing the facet joints responsible for low back pain, mainly by anesthetizing the median branch nerve that innervates the actual joint.

The prevalence of persistent low back pain secondary to the involvement of lumbosacral facet joints has been described in controlled studies as varying from 15% to 45% based on types of population and settings studied.[11,12] Lumbar facet joint interventions are useful in the diagnosis and the therapeutic management of chronic low back pain. Common indications for lumbar diagnostic facet joint interventions are:

- *Somatic or nonradicular low back and/or lower extremity pain*. Duration of pain of at least 3 months with an average pain level of greater than 5 on a scale of 0 to 10. Intermittent or continuous pain causing functional disability, failure to respond to more conservative management, including physical therapy modalities with exercises, chiropractic management, and nonsteroidal antiinflammatory agents, aqua therapy, and medical management.
- *Lack of disc herniation or evidence of radiculitis with no contraindications with understanding of consent, nature of the procedure, needle placement, and sedation*. No history of allergy to contrast administration used, no contraindications or inability to undergo physical therapy, chiropractic management, or inability to tolerate nonsteroidal antiinflammatory medications. Positive response to controlled comparative local anesthetic blocks for therapeutic interventions.

Common contraindications for lumbosacral facet joint interventions are:

- Suspected or proven discogenic, sacroiliac joint, or myofascial pain infection
- Anticoagulant therapy
- Nonaspirin combination antiplatelet therapy
- Pregnancy
- Bleeding diathesis.

PATHOPHYSIOLOGY

Lumbar facet joints have been shown to produce low back and referred lower extremity pain in normal volunteers. Stimulation of lumbar facet joints with injections of hypertonic saline or contrast medium produces back pain and somatic referred pain identical to that commonly seen in patients.[5–9]

This pain also can be relieved by anesthetizing the lumbar facet joints deemed to be responsible for low back pain or the median branch nerve

Disclosure: Consultant for Stryker Corporation & St. Jude Medical Neuro Division.
Space Coast Pain Institute, 595 North Courtenay Parkway, Merritt Island, FL 32953, USA
E-mail address: sgolovac@mac.com

Neuroimag Clin N Am 20 (2010) 203–214
doi:10.1016/j.nic.2010.02.007
1052-5149/10/$ – see front matter © 2010 Elsevier Inc. All rights reserved.

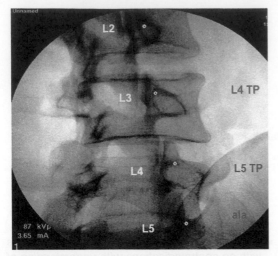

Fig. 1. Oblique view of lumbar target with Scotty dog appearance.

that innervates the joint itself. Pain originating from lumbar facet joints is predominantly present in the low back, buttocks, and thighs; however, it does not follow a reliable segmental pattern. The radiation of referred pain below the knee as far as the foot has been described, but typically pain predominantly involves the proximal parts of the lower extremity.

The prevalence of facet joint pain as a cause of low back pain has been studied extensively but its pathophysiology and diagnosis remains elusive. Lumbar facet joints can be affected by rheumatoid arthritis, osteoarthritis, ankylosing spondylitis, or

ununited epiphyses of the inferior articular processes. The intraoperative reports excising the facet joints have demonstrated changes similar to those of chondromalacia of the patella. Evidence from controlled studies has been unable to establish that facet joint pain is caused by osteoarthritis of facet joints. On plain radiographs, facet joint arthritis appears as commonly in asymptomatic individuals as in patients with back pain. The data from radiological evaluation preclude making the diagnosis of pain of facet joint origin from either plain radiography or computerized tomography (CT) scanning (**Figs. 1** and **2**).

The data also indicate either that osteoarthritis is not a cause of facet joint pain or, when it is, that the pain is caused by some factor other than the simple radiological presence of this condition.[10–16]

Assertions that facet joint arthritis is usually secondary to disc degeneration or spondylosis may not be true, because in approximately 20% of cases facet joint arthritis can be a totally independent disease; and correlation between discogenic pain and facet joint pain or a combination of discogenic and facet joint pain has not been established thus far.

DIAGNOSTIC FACET JOINT BLOCKS

Lumbosacral facet joints can be anesthetized either with intraarticular injection of local anesthetic or by anesthetizing the medial branches of the dorsal rami that innervate the target joint (**Fig. 3**).[17]

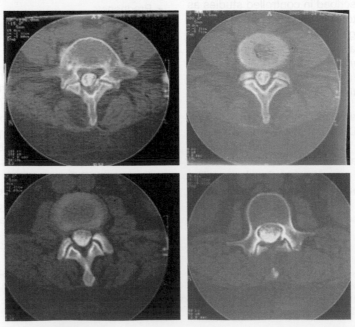

Fig. 2. CT scan, coronal and sagittal views.

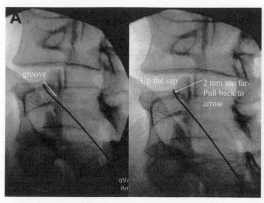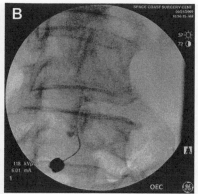

Fig. 3. (A) Radiofrequency ablation needle placement in the groove and up the wall. (B) Below (intraarticular joint injection).

The joint may be considered to be the source of pain if the pain is relieved by joint blockade. It is crucial to follow the required steps to eliminate false-positive responses. True-positive responses may be obtained only by performing controlled blocks. The controlled diagnostic blocks are performed either by placebo injections or by comparative local anesthetic blocks.

Neurophysiologic studies have shown that facet joint capsules contain low-threshold mechanoreceptors, mechanically sensitive nociceptors, and silent nociceptors. The lumbar facet joints have been shown to be capable of being a source of low back pain and referred pain in the lower limbs of normal volunteers (Figs. 4 and 5).

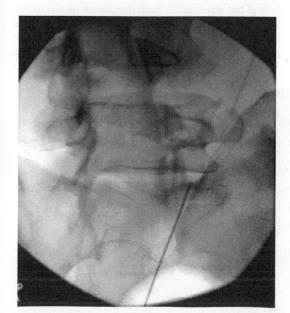

Fig. 4. Dermatomal areas of referred patterns of pain from median branch nerves.

Imaging technologies have not provided valid or reliable means of identifying symptomatic joints. The use of controlled local anesthetic facet joint blocks for the diagnosis of chronic low back pain has been reviewed and validated. Thus, placebo-controlled blocks or comparative local anesthetic blocks using 2 different local anesthetics of differing duration of action on 2 separate occasions, are the only means of confirming the diagnosis of facet joint pain.

Reliability

The face validity of intraarticular facet injections and medial branch blocks has been established by injecting small volumes of local anesthetic into the joint or onto the sensory nerves of the joint. The construct validity of facet joint blocks has been established.

The placebo effect of facet joint injections may be controlled by using strict criteria for determining positive response to controlled anesthetic blocks.

The theory that testing a patient first with lidocaine and subsequently with bupivacaine to identify placebo responders has been tested and proved.[12,14]

Pain provocation response of facet joint injections has been shown to be unreliable. False-positive rates for lumbar facet joint blockade have been reported to be 17% to 49%.[18] The false-negative rate for diagnostic facet joint blocks has been shown to be approximately 8% because of unrecognized intravascular injection of local anesthetic. There is a paucity of literature on the role of therapeutic facet joint blocks. However, facet joint pain may be managed by intraarticular injections, medial branch blocks, or neurolysis of medial branches.[19–21]

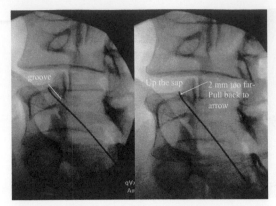

Fig. 5. Oblique view of right L4 median branch nerve needle placement.

Anatomy

The lumbar facet joints are formed by the articulation of the inferior articular process of 1 lumbar vertebra with the superior articular process of the next vertebra. The lumbar joints exhibit the features typical of synovial joints. The articular facets are covered by articular cartilage and a synovial membrane bridges the margins of the articular cartilages of the 2 facets in each joint. Surrounding the synovial membrane is a joint capsule that attaches to the articular processes a short distance beyond the margin of the articular cartilage. Ligaments connect the spinous process, laminae, and bodies of adjacent vertebrae. Anterior and posterior longitudinal ligaments help to stabilize these joints. The articular capsule surrounds facets and allows gliding motion. In the lumbar spine L4/L5 permits most flexion. The anterior longitudinal ligament attaches to anterior bodies and intervertebral discs. It is strong and prevents hyperextension. The posterior longitudinal ligament attaches to posterior bodies and intervertebral discs. It is weaker than the anterior longitudinal ligament and permits hyperflexion.

The ligamentum flava connects adjacent laminae of vertebrae and limits flexion. Intraspinal ligaments connect the spine; these are weak ligaments. Intraspinous ligaments and supraspinous ligaments connect spinous tips. Supraspinous ligaments are stronger than the intraspinous ligament and limit flexion. Intertransverse ligaments connect transverse processes and are weak ligaments.

Innervation

Each lumbar facet joint has dual innervation, being supplied by 2 medial branch nerves. The medial branches are of paramount clinical importance and relevance because they provide sensory innervation to the facet joints. The medial branches of the L1/L4 dorsal rami assume a constant and similar course. Each nerve emerges from its intervertebral foramen and enters the posterior compartment of the back by coursing around the neck of the superior articular process (Fig. 6).

Hugging the neck of the superior articular process, the medial branch passes caudally and slightly dorsally, covered by the mamillo-accessory ligament, hooking medially around the caudal aspect of the root of the superior articular process to enter the multifidus muscle.[22] Intermediate and lateral branches arise from the dorsal ramus at the same point as the medial branch. The medial branch crosses the vertebral lamina where it divides into multiple branches that supply the

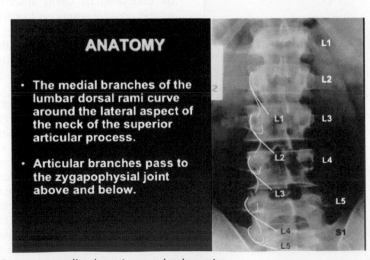

Fig. 6. Anatomy of L1 to L4 median branch nerve lumbar spine.

multifidus muscle, the interspinous muscle and ligament, and 2 facet joints.

The medial branch of the L5 dorsal ramus has a different course and distribution than those of the L1/L4 dorsal rami. Instead of crossing a transverse process, the L5 dorsal ramus crosses the ala of the sacrum. The L5 dorsal ramus is much longer than typical lumbar levels.[22] From the L5/S1 intervertebral foramen, the medial branch of the L5 dorsal ramus runs along the groove formed by the junction of the ala and the root of the superior articular process of the sacrum before hooking medially around the base of the lumbosacral facet joint (Fig. 7).[22]

PROCEDURE

Lumbar facet joint interventions are provided in the form of intraarticular injections, medial branch blocks, and neurolytic blocks. Each procedure is performed by multiple and variable techniques. It is imperative to understand the radiographic/fluoroscopic anatomy (see Fig. 7).

Lumbar Facet Joint Intraarticular Injections

The patient is placed in the prone position on the fluoroscopy table. A towel roll or pillow can be placed under the abdomen to facilitate easier entry into the joint. As with any lumbar intervention, a baseline anterioposterior (AP) fluoroscopic view of the lumbar spine is obtained and the fluoroscope is oriented. Facet joints may or may not be visible on AP fluoroscopy depending on the specific anatomy of the patient (Fig. 8).[23–29]

Fluoroscopic views of the target joint are obtained. The fluoroscopy beam is rotated from the AP view toward the oblique view until the target facet joint is visible. The upper lumbar facet joints are typically aligned toward the sagittal plane and may be visible on AP imaging, whereas the lower joints are typically and increasingly oriented toward the coronal plane so that oblique imaging is necessary to identify joint lines (see Fig. 2).

The target joint is then visualized under fluoroscopic guidance and the skin may be marked. The needle is directed downward and obliquely (from lateral to medial) toward the selected joint under direct fluoroscopic visualization. Contact is made with the inferior articular processes. The needle is then withdrawn slightly and redirected to enter the target facet joint. As the needle is felt to penetrate the joint, advancement is stopped to prevent any potential damage to the articular cartilage.

If there is difficulty in obtaining capsular penetration, access to the articular recesses can be attempted by redirecting the needle just off the margins of the inferior articular processes. Another method of gaining intracapsular entry is to redirect the needle slightly medial or lateral to the posterior joint line so that the needle gains access via its medial placement to the insertion of the capsule on the articular process.

Once the needle is in an appropriate position, 0.2 to 0.5 mL of contrast (eg, iopamidol [Isovue] #200) is then injected into the joint to confirm proper placement. An arthrographic image should then be visualized. During contrast injection, outline of the oval-shaped joint capsule should

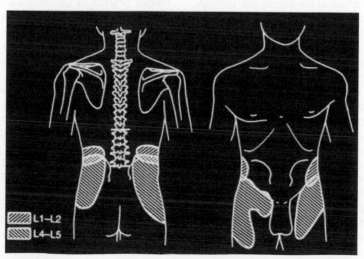

Fig. 7. L5 median branch nerve ablation needle position.

L1–L2
L4–L5

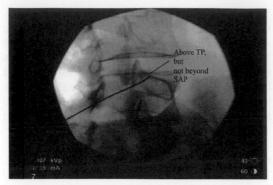

Above TP, but not beyond SAP

107 kVp
mA
60

Fig. 8. Radiofrequency ablation needle placement in the groove and up the wall.

be visualized with lack of vascular uptake and/or epidural spread. After contrast confirmation of intraarticular needle tip placement, the joint is injected with anesthetic agent to complete a diagnostic block, or in combination with a steroid for a therapeutic injection (see **Fig. 3**B).

Medial Branch Blocks

To block the sensory innervation to a lumbar facet joint, it is necessary to block the 2 medial branch nerves that supply the joint. **Box 1** illustrates the nerves to be blocked for each facet joint in the lumbar region. It is simple to remember which nerves need to be blocked to anesthetize a particular joint: block the medial branch at the transverse process at the same level as the joint. Then block the medial branch at the level below the joint. To block the L3/L4 facet joint, block the L2 medial branch at the transverse process of L3 and the L3 medial branch at the transverse process of L4. To block the L5/S1 facet joint, block the L4 medial branch at the L5 transverse process and the L5 dorsal ramus at the sacral ala. Lumbar medial branch blocks have essentially replaced, or should replace, intraarticular injections in the diagnosis of lumbar facet joint pain. Medial branch blocks are easier to perform and safer. Intraarticular injections of lumbar facet joints lack significant therapeutic utility. The joint should only be injected if a patient demonstrates facet sclerosis and performing a radiofrequency procedure is contraindicated either because of a pacemaker or patient refusal. Medial branch blocks have therapeutic utility. There is evidence that medial branch block therapy and radiofrequency neurotomy of lumbar medial branch blocks is effective in managing chronic low back pain.

The posterior primary ramus branch of the exiting segmental nerve divides into lateral and medial branches as soon as it exits from the foramen. The medial branch runs in a dorsal and caudal

---

Box 1
Facet joint level to innervation site

L1/2
  T12 and L1 medial branches
  At L1 transverse process for T12
  At L2 transverse process for L1

L2/3
  L1 and L2 medial branches
  At L2 transverse process for L1
  At L3 transverse process for L2

L3/4
  L2 and L3 medial branches
  At L3 transverse process for L2
  At L4 transverse process for L3

L4/5
  L3 and L4 medial branches
  At L4 transverse process for L3
  At L5 transverse process for L4

L5/S1
  L4 medial branch L5 dorsal ramus
  At L5 transverse process for L4 medial branch
  At sacral ala groove for L5 dorsal ramus

Facet joint nerves to be blocked (medial branches or L5 dorsal ramus)
  Level of transverse process or sacral ala

---

direction to reach the junction of the superior articular processes of the vertebra below the level of the exiting segmental nerve.[20] Therefore, the medial branch of L4 reaches the junction of the L5 processes. This is seen in the lateral view depicting the three-fifths of the superior articular process where the needle tip and shaft should be located to properly dennervate the median branch nerve (**Fig. 9**).

Medial branch block or radiofrequency neurology is performed at this junction between the superior articular and transverse processes. Anatomy may be variable with the target point hidden from sight when an AP projection is used, because the posterior articular process is blocking the view. In some cases access to the target point can only be obtained by using an oblique projection. **Fig. 10** illustrates target points.

Fig. 11 illustrates access to the target point for medial branch block in a lateral projection. For L5 dorsal ramus block, the junction between the sacral articular process and upper sacral border

TARGET ZONES

Ventrally the neural foramen can be inadvertently entered

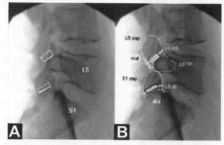

Fig. 9. Lateral view of needle placement, denoting bone in front of needle (*A, B*).

where L5 dorsal ramus runs, there is no pedicle to serve as a radiological landmark. **Fig. 12** shows the target point for L5 dorsal ramus block in an anatomic illustration.

Prone Position: Oblique

The patient is placed in the prone position with a pillow under the abdomen. Fluoroscopic imaging is obtained. The C-arm must be adjusted to an oblique position. To maximally visualize the landmarks of the Scotty dog configuration, an approximate 25° to 30° angle is necessary depending on the specific level from L1 to L4 medial branches (**Fig. 13**).

The needle is advanced toward the dorsal aspect of the root of the transverse process to ensure safe needle depth away from the ventral ramus. Using an oblique view with the Scotty dog identified, the needle is advanced down the beam toward the target using a slightly superior starting position to the final target (see **Fig. 1**).

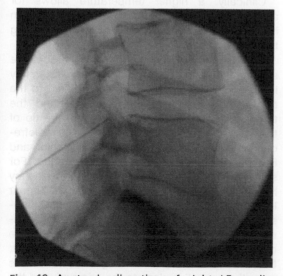

Fig. 10. Anatomic dissection of right L5 median branch nerve.

The needle needs to be directed anterior, medial, and caudal to reach the target location, using a Scotty dog view. Needles are typically placed down to contact with the bony end point using oblique fluoroscopic imaging. Before injection, however, final needle tip position should be confirmed using AP and lateral imaging to ensure that the needle tip is neither too deep nor too medial, or by arthrography. On AP imaging, the tip of the needle should be at least in line with the lateral margin of the silhouette of the superior articular process and, if possible, medial to this margin.

On lateral imaging, the needle tip should be within the confines of the shadow of the dorsal elements and not protruding into the foramen. The superior articular process frequently bulges laterally, overlapping the target point dorsally. If the needle appears lateral to this point, it has contacted a thick transverse process instead of the superior articular process. In this case, the needle usually needs to be adjusted dorsally until the correct position is obtained on AP and oblique or lateral views. Before injection, the bevel opening should be medial and slightly inferior to reduce lateral and superior flow to the intervertebral foramen, especially if the needle is inadvertently placed higher than the target position (see **Fig. 9**).

Prone Position: AP

The patient is positioned in the prone position with a pillow under the abdomen. Fluoroscopic imaging is obtained. The C-arm must be adjusted straight AP from the skin entry point laterally using posteroanterior (PA) imaging which is usually just above the tip of the target transverse process.

As shown in **Fig. 6** in PA projection, there is a clear double contour in the caudal end plate of L4. With axial rotation of the C-arm in the sagittal plane, the angle in the sagittal plane is changed to eliminate the double contour in the L4 end plate.[30,31] The needle is advanced toward the

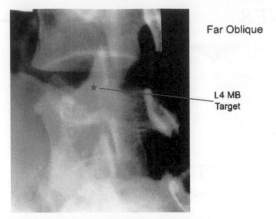

Far Oblique

L4 MB
Target

Fig. 11. Target of left median branch nerve.

back of the root of the transverse process to ensure safe needle depth away from the ventral ramus (see **Fig. 11**). The needle is directed anterior, medial, and caudal to reach the target location (see **Fig. 11**). On AP imaging, the tip of the needle should be at least in line with the lateral margin of the silhouette of the superior articular process and, if possible, medial to this margin. The superior articular process frequently bulges laterally, overlapping the target point dorsally. If the needle appears lateral to this point, it has contacted a thick transverse process instead of the superior articular process. In this case, the needle usually needs to be adjusted dorsally until the correct position is obtained. Before injection, the bevel opening should be medial and slightly inferior to reduce lateral and superior flow to the intervertebral foramen, especially if the needle is inadvertently placed higher than the target position.

L5 Dorsal Ramus Blocks

Position the patient in the prone position with a pillow under the abdomen. Begin with an AP

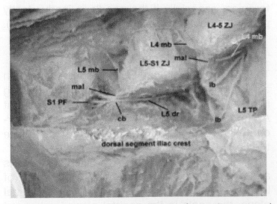

Fig. 12. Needle comparison of size of actual nerve and reference to proximity of needle required to ablate nerves.

view of the L5/S1 segment (see **Fig. 7**). Rotate the fluoroscope approximately 10° to 15° oblique toward the side to be blocked to view the junction of the sacral ala and the superior articular process of S1. Further obliquity usually places the medial iliac crest in front of the trajectory to the target position. If the ilium obscures the view of the target point as the C-arm is rotated obliquely, cephalad tilt of the C-arm usually brings the target into clear view by moving the ilium caudad within the fluoroscopic image. An angled needle tip allows for adequate steering of the needle to the target despite a cephalad to caudad needle trajectory. Once a clear path to the target point for the L5 dorsal ramus is identified, a skin insertion point is chosen. The target point is recognized as a notch between the sacral ala and the superior articulating process of S1. The target point lies opposite the middle of the base of the superior articular process and thus slightly below the silhouette at the top of the sacral ala. Higher placement is associated with spread into the L5/S1 epidural space and lower placement with spread to the S1 posterior sacral foramina. The needle is advanced directly down the beam to the target position.

Radiofrequency Neurotomy

Radiofrequency lesioning is performed using either a heat lesion or pulsed mode radiofrequency. A thermal radiofrequency neurotomy lesion for facet denervation is performed at 80° to 85°C for 60 seconds. Two sites along the superior articulating process need to be treated to ensure that the median branch nerve has been treated.

Clinically, a higher temperature allows for a larger lesion to be made. The size of the lesion is influenced by the vascularity of the surrounding tissue.

The greater the vascularity of the tissue, the smaller the lesion. Pulsed mode radiofrequency is an application of a strong electric field to the tissue that surrounds the electrode and the temperature of the tissue surrounding the tip of the electrode does not exceed 42°C. The radiofrequency current is applied in a pulsed fashion and heat is dissipated during the silent period. For safe and accurate conventional radiofrequency heat lesioning, the medial branch at typical lumbar levels is accessible for only a limited length opposite the middle two-fourths of the neck of the superior articular process.[32] Distal to this area, the nerve lies under the mamillo-accessory ligament; this is not amenable to lesioning. Proximal to this area, the nerve lies close to the origin of, and the proximal course of, the intermediate and lateral

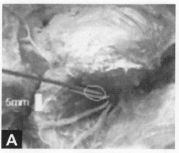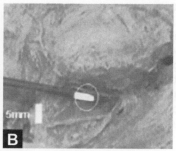

Parallel to nerve- different needle sizes

Fig. 13. Lateral three-fifths view of needle placement (*A, B*).

branches of the dorsal ramus, thus, these branches may be lesioned.

The target point for placement of the electrode is the lateral surface of the superior articular surface just above its junction with the root of the transverse process. In lateral view, this portion of the superior articular surface is relatively narrow. This area is referred to as the neck of the superior articular process. The target nerve runs across this neck, from the intervertebral foramen to where it hooks medially under the mamillo-accessory ligament.[20,22–30,33,34] The objective in radiofrequency is to target the nerve. The appropriate target zone is approximately the central two-thirds or central two-fourths of the neck.

Appropriate preparation is performed. PA view or oblique view needles are positioned similar to the descriptions for medial branch blocks. For radiofrequency thermoneurolysis with a heat lesion, the cannula is placed along the course of the medial branch or at the L5 level on the posterior primary ramus (see **Fig. 12**).

The number of lesions required to coagulate the target nerve depends on the size of the tip of the electrode and the relative size of the superior articular process. Various considerations apply to the trajectory of the electrode. At all segmental levels, the electrode needs to run parallel to the nerve. From lumbar levels L1 to L4 medial branches, the electrode is positioned oblique to the sagittal plane. For all nerves, it is crucial that the electrode is placed as closely as possible, parallel to the course of the nerve to maximize the lesioning of the affected nerve targeted (see **Fig. 12**; **Fig. 14**).

RELATIVE CONTRAINDICATIONS

Relative contraindications to interventional techniques have been described in patients receiving treatment with nonsteroidal antiinflammatory medications (especially aspirin), because of concerns that these agents may compromise coagulation.[35] Dreyfuss and colleagues[36] have provided a detailed description of the role of anticoagulants in interventional pain management. Nonetheless, discontinuation of nonsteroidal antiinflammatory drugs and aspirin is recommended before lumbar facet joint intervention techniques. Before lumbar facet joint interventions, patients on warfarin therapy should have their prothrombin time checked and documented to be at acceptable levels. In stopping anticoagulant therapy, the risk/benefit ratio of the procedure should be considered.

In addition, the pain physician may consult with the physician in charge of anticoagulant therapy. It is prudent to advise the patient to contact the physician in charge of anticoagulant therapy and let them make the decision as to the

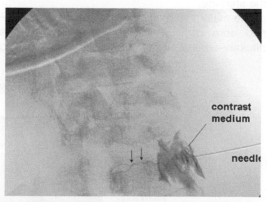

Fig. 14. Intraarterial injection of a radicular feeder artery in the cervical spine during a transforaminal injection during subdigital angiography.

appropriateness of discontinuation of anticoagulant therapy. Aspirin and nonsteroidal antiinflammatory drugs alone are considered safe. Combination of these drugs or other antiplatelet therapy with clopidogrel (Plavix) or ticlopidine HCL (Ticlid) may be considered to increase the risk of spinal hematoma. The risk and potential discontinuation may be considered by the physician in charge of antiplatelet therapy.

SIDE EFFECTS AND COMPLICATIONS

Complications from facet joint nerve blocks or intraarticular injections in the lumbar spine are exceedingly rare.[37–40]

The most common complications of intraarticular injections and medial branch blocks are twofold:

1. Complications related to the administration of various drugs. Most problems such as local swelling, pain at the site of the needle insertion, and pain in the low back are short-lived and self-limited.
2. More serious complications may include dural puncture, spinal cord trauma, subdural injection, neural trauma, injection into the intervertebral foramen, and hematoma formation; infectious complications including epidural abscess and bacterial meningitis; and side effects related to the administration of steroids, local anesthetics, and other drugs.[32,41–47]

Table 1 lists potential complications of lumbar facet joint interventions.

Minor complications include lightheadedness, flushing, sweating, nausea, hypotension, syncope, pain at the injection site as described earlier, and nonpostural headaches. Side effects related to the administration of steroids are generally attributed to the chemistry or to the pharmacology of the steroids.

The major theoretic complications of corticosteroid administration include suppression of the pituitary-adrenal axis, hypocorticism, Cushing

Table 1	
Potential complications of lumbar facet joint interventions	
Pain	**At Site of Needle Insertion**
Bleeding	Soft tissue hematoma Epidural hematoma Spinal cord hematoma Nerve root sheath hematoma
Trauma	Inadvertent injection Dural puncture Subdural injection Epidural injection Foraminal injection Intravascular injection
Radiofrequency	Nerve root ablation Spinal cord ablation Dysesthesias Allodynia
Infection	Soft tissue abscess Epidural abscess Facet joint abscess Meningitis Encephalitis
Hypoesthesia	

syndrome, osteoporosis, avascular necrosis of bone, steroid myopathy, epidural lipomatosis, weight gain, fluid retention, and hyperglycemia. Evaluation of the effect of neuraxial steroids on weight and bone mass density showed no significant differences in patients undergoing various types of interventional techniques with or without steroids.[48] Reported complications of radiofrequency thermoneurolysis include a worsening of the usual pain, burning or dysesthesias, decreased sensation and allodynia in the paravertebral skin or the facets denervated, transient leg pain, persistent leg weakness, and inadvertent lesioning of the spinal nerve or ventral ramus resulting in motor deficits, sensory loss, and possible deafferentation

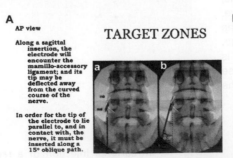
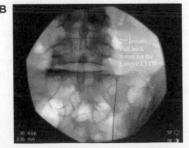

A AP view

TARGET ZONES

Along a sagittal insertion, the electrode will encounter the mamillo-accessory ligament; and its tip may be deflected away from the curved course of the nerve.

In order for the tip of the electrode to lie parallel to, and in contact with, the nerve, it must be inserted along a 15° oblique path.

Fig. 15. (*A*) Needle breeches up to the L4 vertebra and the single needle placement on the right (*B*) needle is located at the L5 median branch nerve.

pain. A spinal cord lesion can lead to paraplegia, loss of motor, proprioception and sensory function, bowel and bladder dysfunction, Brown-Séquard syndrome, and spinal cord infarction. Intravascular injections can lead to a disaster (**Fig. 15**).

As long as the necessary steps are followed and the correct precautions taken in performing a radiofrequency ablation, overall improvement should be noticed by the patient within 10 to 14 days. Exercise, physical therapy, and improvement in body mechanics are essential to maximize outcomes and pain relief.

REFERENCES

1. Goldthwait JE. The lumbosacral articulation: an explanation of many cases of lumbago, sciatica, and paraplegia. Boston Med Surg J 1911;164:365–72.
2. Ghormley RK. Low back pain. With special reference to the articular facets, with presentation of an operative procedure. JAMA 1933;101:1773–7.
3. Badgley CE. The articular facets in relation to low back pain and sciatic radiation. J Bone Joint Surg 1941;23:481.
4. Hirsch D, Inglemark B, Miller M. The anatomical basis for low back pain. Acta Orthop Scand 1963; 33:1–17.
5. McCall IW, Park WM, O'Brien JP. Induced pain referral from posterior elements in normal subjects. Spine 1979;4:441–6.
6. Marks R. Distribution of pain provoked from lumbar facet joints and related structures during diagnostic spinal infiltration. Pain 1989;39:37–40.
7. Fukui S, Ohseto K, Shiotani M, et al. Distribution of referral pain from the lumbar zygapophyseal joints and dorsal rami. Clin J Pain 1997;13:303–7.
8. Windsor RE, King FJ, Roman SJ, et al. Electrical stimulation induced lumbar medial branch referral patterns. Pain Physician 2002;5:347–54.
9. Dreyfuss P, Schwarzer AC, Lau P, et al. Specificity of lumbar medial branch and L5 dorsal ramus blocks: a computed tomography study. Spine (Phila Pa 1976) 1997;22:895–902.
10. Bogduk N, Dreyfuss P, Govind J. A narrative review of lumbar medial branch neurotomy for the treatment of back pain. Pain Med 2009;10(6):1035–45.
11. Schwarzer AC, Wang S, Bogduk N, et al. Prevalence and clinical features of lumbar zygapophysial joint pain. A study in an Australian population with chronic low back pain. Am Rheum Dis 1995;54: 100–6.
12. Bogduk N. International spinal injection society guidelines for the performance of spinal injection procedures. Part 1: zygapophysial joint blocks. Clin J Pain 1997;13:285–302.
13. Schwarzer AC, Aprill CN, Derby R, et al. Clinical features of patients with pain stemming from the lumbar zygapophysial joints. Is the lumbar facet syndrome a clinical entity? Spine 1994;19: 1132–7.
14. Boswell MV, Singh V, Staats PS, et al. Accuracy of precision diagnostic blocks in the diagnosis of chronic spinal pain of facet or zygapophysial joint origin. Pain Physician 2003;6:449–56.
15. Schwarzer AC, Wang SC, O'Driscoll D, et al. The ability of computed tomography to identify a painful zygapophysial joint in patients with chronic low back pain. Spine 1995;20:907–12.
16. Magora A, Bigos SJ, Stolov WC, et al. The significance of medical imaging findings in low back pain. Pain Clinic 1994;7:99–105.
17. Schwarzer AC, Derby R, Aprill CN, et al. The value of the provocation response in lumbar zygapophysial joint injections. Clin J Pain 1994;10:309–13.
18. Sehgal N, Dunbar EE, Shah RV, et al. Systematic review of diagnostic utility of facet (zygapophysial) joint injections in chronic spinal pain: an update. Pain Physician 2007;10:213–28.
19. Schwarzer AC, Aprill CN, Derby R, et al. The false-positive rate of uncontrolled diagnostic blocks of the lumbar zygapophysial joints. Pain 1994;58: 195–200.
20. Boswell MV, Trescot AM, Datta S, et al. Interventional techniques: evidence-based practice guidelines in the management of chronic spinal pain. Pain Physician 2007;10:7–111.
21. Boswell MV, Colson JD, Sehgal N, et al. A systematic review 276 interventional techniques in chronic spinal pain of therapeutic facet joint interventions in chronic spinal pain. Pain Physician 2007;10:229–53.
22. Carette S, Marcoux S, Truchon R, et al. A controlled trial of corticosteroid injections into facet joints for chronic low back pain. N Engl J Med 1991;325: 1002–7.
23. Fuchs S, Erbe T, Fischer HL, et al. Intraarticular hyaluronic acid versus glucocorticoid injections for nonradicular pain in the lumbar spine. J Vasc Interv Radiol 2005;16:1493–8.
24. Schulte TL, Pietila TA, Heidenreich J, et al. Injection therapy of lumbar facet syndrome: a prospective study. Acta Neurochir (Wien) 2006;148:1165–72.
25. Lynch MC, Taylor JF. Facet joint injection for low back pain. A clinical study. J Bone Joint Surg Br 1986;68:138–41.
26. Murtagh FR. Computed tomography and fluoroscopy guided anesthesia and steroid injection in facet syndrome. Spine 1988;13:686–9.
27. Destouet JM, Gilula LA, Murphy WA, et al. Lumbar facet joint injection: indication, technique, clinical correlation, and preliminary results. Radiology 1982;145:321–5.
28. Lippitt AB. The facet joint and its role in spine pain. Management with facet joint injections. Spine 1984; 9:746–50.

29. Lau LS, Littlejohn GO, Miller MH. Clinical evaluation of intraarticular injections for lumbar facet joint pain. Med J Aust 1985;143:563–5.

30. Boswell MV, Colson JD, Sehgal N, et al. A systematic review of therapeutic facet joint interventions in chronic spinal pain. Pain Physician 2007;10:229–53.

31. Lau P, Mercer S, Govind J, et al. The surgical anatomy of lumbar medial branch neurotomy (facet denervation). Pain Med 2004;5:289–98.

32. Martinez-Suarez JE, Camblor L, Salva S, et al. Thermocoagulation of lumbar facet joints. Experience in 252 patients. Rev Soc Esp Dolor 2005;12:425–8.

33. Cavanaugh JM, Lu Y, Chen C, et al. Pain generation in lumbar and cervical facet joints. J Bone Joint Surg Am 2006;2:63–7.

34. Niemistö L, Kalso E, Malmivaara A, et al. Cochrane Collaboration Back Review Group. Radiofrequency denervation for neck and back pain: a systematic review within the framework of the Cochrane Collaboration Back Review Group. Spine 2003;28:1877–88.

35. van Kleef M, Barendse GA, Kessels A, et al. Randomized trial of radiofrequency lumbar facet denervation for chronic low back pain. Spine (Phila Pa 1976) 1999;24:1937–42.

36. Dreyfuss P, Halbrook B, Pauza K, Joshi A, et al. Efficacy and validity of radiofrequency neurotomy for chronic lumbar zygapophysial joint pain. Spine (Phila Pa 1976) 2000;25:1270–7.

37. Schofferman J, Kine G. Effectiveness of repeated radiofrequency neurotomy for lumbar facet pain. Spine 2004;29:2471–3.

38. Vad V, Cano W, Basrai D, et al. Role of radiofrequency denervation in lumbar zygapophyseal joint synovitis in baseball pitchers: a clinical experience. Pain Physician 2003;6:307–12.

39. Mogalles AA, Dreval' ON, Akatov OV, et al. Percutaneous laser denervation of the zygapophyseal joints in the pain facet syndrome. Zh Vopr Neirokhir Im N N Burdenko 2004;1:20–5.

40. North RB, Han M, Zahurak M, et al. Radiofrequency lumbar facet denervation: analysis of prognostic factors. Pain 1994;57:77–83.

41. Tzaan WC, Tasker RR. Percutaneous radiofrequency facet rhizotomy experience with 118 procedures and reappraisal of its value. Can J Neurol Sci 2000;27:125–30.

42. Schaerer JP. Radiofrequency facet rhizotomy in the treatment of chronic neck and low back pain. Int Surg 1978;63:53–9.

43. Birkenmaier C, Veihelmann A, Trouillier H, et al. Percutaneous cryodenervation of lumbar facet joints: a prospective clinical trial. Int Orthop 2007; 31(4):525–30.

44. Staender M, Maerz U, Tonn JC, et al. Computerized tomography-guided kryorhizotomy in 76 patients with lumbar facet joint syndrome. J Neurosurg Spine 2005;3:444–9.

45. Sluijter ME. The lumbar medial branch. In: Radiofrequency. Part 1: the lumbo-sacral region. Switzerland: Flivo Press; 2001. p. 105–18.

46. Dreyfuss P, Kaplan M, Dreyer SJ. Zygapophyseal joint injection techniques in the spinal axis. In: Lennard TA, editor. Pain procedures in clinical practice. 2nd edition. Philadelphia: Hanley & Belfus, Inc; 2000. p. 276–308.

47. Raj PP, Shah RV, Kaye AD, et al. Bleeding risk in interventional pain practice: assessment, management, and review of the literature. Pain Physician 2004;7:3–51.

48. Horlocker TT, Wedel DJ, Benzon H, et al. Regional anesthesia in the anticoagulated patient: defining the risks (the second ASRA consensus conference on neuraxial anesthesia and anticoagulation). Reg Anesth Pain Med 2003;28:172–97.

Pharmaceuticals Used in Image-Guided Spine Interventions

John M. Mathis, MD, MSc[a],*, Stanley Golovac, MD[b],
Charles H. Cho, MD, MBA[c]

KEYWORDS

- Image-guided spine interventions
- Epidural steroid injections • Spine pain management
- Vertebroplasty • Bone cements • Steroids • Anesthetics

CORTICOSTEROIDS

Corticosteroids have a long history in the treatment of pain related to spine disease, having been used since the 1960s.[1] They were originally injected epidurally and intrathecally for pain management. By the 1980s, there were reports of complications that included arachnoiditis, meningitis, and paraparesis/paraplegia.[2,3] Controversy was sufficient in Australia that an explicit government warning was issued about the use of corticosteroids for epidural pain management.[4] Review of the scientific literature regarding these findings revealed that many of the complications resulted from the intrathecal use of corticosteroids.[2–6] It is now known that definite side effects can result from these drugs, and physicians should be aware of these side effects and include potential complications in their explanations to their patients.

Corticosteroids are believed to produce chemical stabilization of the local environment, which can produce pain relief by reducing the local amount of phospholipase A2 and arachidonic acid, as well as decreasing the cell-mediated inflammatory and immunologic responses.[1] The usual dosages of various steroids for epidural steroid injections are given in **Table 1**. Dose equivalents are given in **Table 2**.

The most common corticosteroid used for spine injections has been a long-acting form of methylprednisolone acetate (Depo-Medrol, Pharmacia-Upjohn, Chesterfield, MO, USA). This drug is available in 40- and 80- mg/mL doses. The acetate formulation is quite insoluble in water and has a long half-life in tissues. It has a relative strength of approximately 5 times that of hydrocortisone and often contains the preservative polyethylene glycol, which is thought to be potentially neurotoxic. Indeed, this material may be the cause of arachnoiditis if given into the intrathecal space. Depo-Medrol is a particulate mixture and can create stroke if injected intra-arterially (ie, into a radicular spinal artery during an attempted cervical foraminal injection). The particulate nature is increased by adding anesthetic solutions, as the combination increases precipitation within the syringe. Mixing Depo-Medrol with anesthetic in the same syringe is contraindicated on the package insert.

Another option for an injectable corticosteroid is the combination of betamethasone sodium phosphate and betamethasone acetate (Celestone

Disclosures Mathis: Industry/Government connections: Consultant, Food and Drug Administration-Orthopedics and Rehabilitation Division (Washington, DC), Orthovita (Malvern, PA), Biomimetics (Nashville, TN), Crosstrees Medical (Denver, CO).
Disclosures CHO: No disclosure. No industry affiliation or industry grants.
[a] Centers for Advanced Imaging, Roanoke, VA 24014, USA
[b] St. Jude Medical Neuro Division, 595 North Courtenay Parkway, Merritt Island, FL 32953, USA
[c] Department of Radiology, Brigham and Women's Hospital and Harvard Medical School, 75 Francis Street, Boston, MA, USA
* Corresponding author.
E-mail address: jmathis@rev.net

Table 1
Recommended dosages of typical steroid preparations used in epidural steroid injections

Steroid	Dose (mg)
Depo-Medrol	40–80
Kenalog	40–80
Celestone	6–12
Dexamethasone	6–12

Soluspan, Schering, Kentworth, NJ, USA). This combines a short- and long-acting form of betamethasone in the same injectable solution. It contains no preservative and comes in 6mg/mL doses. Betamethasone has approximately 30 times the strength of hydrocortisone. It seems to have a lesser particulate nature and a decreased tendency to precipitate when mixed with anesthetics. All of these properties make it less apt to create arachnoiditis when injected intrathecally. Because there were periods when the availability of Depo-Medrol and Celestone was decreased, some labs used a long-acting form of triamcinolone (Kenalog,
Bristol-Myers Squibb, New York, NY, USA).[7] This material is also particulate (similar to Depo-Medrol) and contains the preservative polyethylene glycol. It is available in a 40-mg/mL dosage and has approximately 5 times the strength of hydrocortisone. It seems to be equivalent to Depo-Medrol with no discernable advantages and is recommended in the same dosage as Depo-Medrol (80 mg).

The stroke potential of each of these corticosteroids is related to their particulate nature. With Depo-Medrol and Kenalog, the particulate nature is made worse by mixing with anesthetic in the injection syringe. This seems to be a smaller problem with Celestone. However, all 3 are

particulate and may produce stroke if injected intra-arterially.

Dexamethasone sodium phosphate has been substituted for the above-mentioned corticosteroids with the intent of avoiding the potential for stroke (with inadvertent intra-arterial injection). It is approved for intravenous injection but not for intra-arterial injection. Dexamethasone also contains a preservative (benzyl alcohol),which makes it particulate. Derby and colleagues[8] found that particles of dexamethasone are approximately one-tenth the size of a red blood cell and did not aggregate when mixed with lidocaine. There is no direct proof that using dexamethasone instead of other corticosteroids prevents stroke, although it does seem to give an additional margin of safety with respect to particle size and aggregation.

ANESTHETIC AGENTS

Local anesthetic agents are commonly added as part of the injectate used for numerous spinal and pain management injection procedures.[1] Local anesthetics are sodium channel–blocking drugs that can halt electrical impulse conduction in peripheral nerves, spinal roots, and autonomic ganglia.[9] To block nerve conduction, the local anesthetic must cover at least 3 consecutive sodium channels (nodes of Ranvier) (**Fig. 1**). Binding to the sodium channel interrupts nerve impulse transmission. The binding is reversible (reversibility varying with the length of action of each anesthetic). Differential blocking occurs

Table 2
Approximate equivalent glucocorticoid dosages

Drug	Equivalent Dose (mg)
Cortisone	30
Hydrocortisone	25
Prednisone	6
Prednisolone	6
Methylprednisolone	5
Triamcinolone	5
Dexamethasone	1
Betamethasone	1

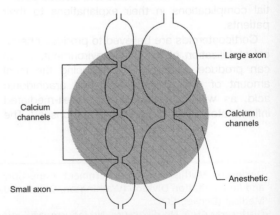

Fig. 1. This line drawing diagrammatically shows a small and large nerve adjacent to each other. A representative anesthetic injection may cover more calcium channels (nodes of Ranvier) in the small nerve than in the large nerve within the same relative volume. This allows differential blockage of pain (smallest), sensory (intermediate), and motor (largest) nerve fibers.

because fibers carrying different types of information (pain, sensory, motor) are of different sizes. The smallest of these are the nociceptive (pain) fibers. These fibers experience calcium channel blockade with the smallest amount of anesthetic because a physically small amount of material spreads sufficiently far enough to cover 3 small sodium channel (nociceptive) receptors, whereas that amount may not adequately cover 3 larger receptors (sensory or motor). Progressively larger fibers require a larger volume of anesthetic to produce coverage that will block enough adjacent channels to stop conduction. This means that pain fibers are the most sensitive, followed by sensory fibers and then motor fibers, allowing the potential for pain relief without obligatory motor blockade.

Local anesthetics are organic amines, with an intermediary ester or amide linkage separating the lipophilic ringed head from the hydrophilic hydrocarbon tail. The amino-ester group of anesthetics includes members such as procaine, tetracaine, and benzocaine. These anesthetics have been used for a long time and are known to have a higher allergic potential than the amide-linked group of anesthetics (lidocaine, bupivacaine, and ropivacaine) now in common usage.[10] The amino-ester group of anesthetics is thought to have allergic potential because of the metabolite para-aminobenzoic acid (PABA). The amide group of anesthetics does not have this metabolite and is known to have a very low allergic potential and little cross-reactivity. However, the amide group may contain the preservative methylparaben. This compound is metabolized to PABA and can produce cross-reactivity for potential allergic reactions with the ester group of anesthetics. Preservative-free amide anesthetics are therefore recommended for all injection procedures.

Lidocaine represented a common first-generation member of the amide anesthetic group. It is considered to be safe except in large quantities that generally exceeded 500 mg. It has a relatively short duration of action usually lasting only several hours. Bupivacaine is a second-generation amide anesthetic that has a prolonged duration of action. It is, however, associated with cardiac and neurotoxic reactions and has a maximum recommended safe dose of 150 mg.[11] Because of the poorer cardiac profile of bupivacaine that resulted from long-term sodium channel blockade in heart muscle, third-generation amide anesthetics were developed. Ropivacaine is a member of this group and produces local anesthesia for a longer period like bupivacaine but with a better cardiac profile.[12] Injections of local anesthetic in percutaneous spine interventions are small enough that one

should generally never approach the maximum allowable dosages.

Bupivacaine and ropivacaine come in different concentrations (0.25%, 0.5%, and 0.75% and 0.2% and 0.5%, respectively). The lower dosages are useful for pain relief in epidural and nerve blockage injections. The more-concentrated dosages produce motor blockade, which is an unwanted side effect with these procedures. The amounts of these drugs used in outpatient, percutaneous procedures are small compared with that needed to produce cardiac or neurotoxic effects.

ANTIBIOTICS

Antibiotics are needed only for selected procedures in spine intervention. These include discography, intradiscal electrothermal therapy, percutaneous discectomy, vertebroplasty and kyphoplasty, implantable pumps, and stimulators.[1] Most routine injection procedures do not require antibiotics. The purpose of antibiotic coverage in most of these procedures is to decrease the chance of seeding bacteria in poorly vascularized sites, such as the disk or around foreign bodies (implantables). The antibiotics used for these procedures are generally not the more toxic or sophisticated ones, from the infectious disease standpoint. As penicillin allergy is not uncommon, a broad-spectrum antibiotic with minimal or no penicillin cross-reactivity is generally chosen. Cephalosporins have minimal penicillin cross-reactivity, and therefore a reasonable choice is _cefazolin (Ancef). Cefazolin is the most common antibiotic used for this purpose[13] and is given in a 1-g dosage (intravenously [IV] or intramuscularly [IM]) 30 minutes before the procedure. In addition, it can be added to the contrast for discography procedures (usually 20–100 mg, with the upper range used when no IV antibiotics are given). It must be born in mind that this antibiotic will cause grand mal seizure activity if given intrathecally.[14] No antibiotic should be included if a transdural approach is used.

In some patients, allergy or lack of access to an IV may make alternate choices better. Another commonly used antibiotic in the interventional laboratory is ciprofloxacin (Cipro). This is a fluoroquinolone with a broad spectrum of coverage and without cross-reactivity to penicillin. It is usually given orally in dosages of 500 mg twice a day. It can be given IV (400 mg) but must be given slowly over a prolonged period to avoid pain and IV site reaction. This generally limits its use in the laboratory to oral administration.

Another good alternative is levofloxacin (Levaquin), which is a fluorinated carboxyquinolone. It may be given orally or IV and has similar plasma and time profiles for both routes of administration, making it a good choice for either route (again, slow administration is required when given IV). The general dosage is 500 mg every 24 hours.

ANALGESICS

Conscious sedation may be needed with a few procedures in the realm of image-guided spine pain management (eg, percutaneous vertebroplasty). It works fine for the duration the patient is on the table.[1] However, as some procedures are frankly painful (eg, discography) and others associated with a postprocedure pain flair (eg, epidural steroid injection), one may need to administer or prescribe analgesics that are appropriate for the patients' pain level and suspected duration.[15] These analgesics need not be administered long-term. The mainstay of postprocedural pain management is an opioid, nonsteroidal antiinflammatory (NSAID), or a combination drug that contains both.

Mild to intermediate pain may be managed by the use of NSAIDs alone or in combination with a weak opioid (eg, codeine, hydrocodone, dihydrocodeine, oxycodone). Controlled trials show little difference in efficacy of the NSAID category, and therefore, it is usually sufficient to find one that works.[16] There is potential toxicity from the NSAIDs to the gastrointestinal, genitourinary, central nervous, and hematologic systems. One should consider avoiding NSAIDs in patients who are predisposed to developing gastropathy or bleeding diathesis. Ketorolac (Toradol) is very effective for short-term use in intermediate pain relief.[17] It is recommended only for short-term use and should be administered with an initial loading dose given IV or IM before oral dosing. Multidose administration (IV or IM) is as follows: (1) for patients younger than 65 years, 30 mg every 6 hours, not to exceed 120 mg and (2) for patients older than 65 years, patients with renal impairment, and those weighing less than 50 kg, 15 mg every 6 hours, not to exceed 60 mg. If there is breakthrough pain, one should not increase the dosage but should add additional analgesic coverage. Regular, rather than intermittent, therapy promotes both antiinflammatory and analgesic effects.

Intermediate pain is often managed with the weaker opioids such as codeine, hydrocodone, dihydrocodeine, or oxycodone. These drugs are usually formulated as combination products and are considered weak only in so far as the inclusion of aspirin, acetaminophen, or ibuprofen results in a ceiling dose above which the incidence of toxicity increases. Prescribed alone, some of these drugs can manage even severe pain. Codeine is emetogenic and is prescribed to a much lesser extent than in the past. Hydrocodone preparations (ie, Vicodin, Lortab) are now more commonly used. The potency of hydrocodone is between that of codeine and oxycodone. It is not available as a single-entity preparation. Oxycodone, now available as a combination product (eg, Percocet, Percodan) and as a single-entity preparation (eg, Roxicodone, Percodan), is very effective. It is also now available in a very potent, slow-release formulation (OxyContin).

The most potent opioids are reserved for severe pain (ie, intractable pain associated with cancer). The members of this group include morphine, controlled-release morphine (MS Contin), hydromorphone (Dilaudid), meperidine (Demerol), and methadone (Dolophine). Although previously discussed, oxycodone falls somewhat within this category when used as a single-entity preparation.

Most interventional radiologists do not prescribe these more-potent drugs. However, if your practice includes this type of therapy, a careful study and detailed understanding of these drugs is necessary. Good documentation of their need and use is also key.

ADJUVANT ANALGESICS

Classic pain is usually well handled by one of the NSAIDs, an opioid, or a combination product.[1] These analgesics effectively deal with pain resulting from classic nociceptors that respond to intense, potentially tissue-damaging stimuli. However, neuropathic pain results from spontaneous discharge of injured nerves. It may be enhanced by sympathetic afferent activity as well. This type of pain is not easy to control with standard analgesics, and successful treatment has been achieved when using adjuvant drugs such as antidepressants and anticonvulsants.[18]

When neuropathic pain is described as burning and constant, the tricyclic antidepressants become the first line of therapy. Syndromes such as posttherapeutic neuralgia and phantom limb pain are examples. Amitriptyline (Elavil) is the most studied drug used for this type of dysesthetic pain.[19] The operative mechanism for antidepressant-mediated analgesia is believed to be associated with increased circulating pools of norepinephrine and serotonin created by reductions in the postsynaptic uptake of these neurotransmitters. The quantities of drug administered are well below that needed to relieve depression and suggest a separate mechanism of action.

When neuropathic pain is described as intermittent but sharp and lancinating, anticonvulsant drugs have been used with success and tried before the antidepressants. It is believed that they relieve pain by dampening ectopic foci of electrical activity and spontaneous discharge from injured nerves. Although carbamazepine and phenytoin have been useful as adjuvant analgesics, gabapentin (Neurontin) is a new anticonvulsant that has been found to be effective for neuropathic pain relief while avoiding most of the side effects found with the other anticonvulsants.[20]

These and other adjuvant analgesics should be known and used when neuropathic pain contributes to the patient's discomfort.

RADIOGRAPHIC CONTRAST

Numerous choices exist for a radiographic contrast agent used in minimally invasive spine procedures.[1] The main concern is related to the allergic potential and use within the thecal sac. There is no method to completely avoid the potential for allergy. Premedication is indicated in all patients with known allergy or prior reaction. If that reaction is severe then iodinated contrast use should be fully avoided. Substitution of another type of material may be useful (ie, gadolinium).[21] Pretreatment should include corticosteroids (prednisone, 50 mg by mouth, 3 to 4 times beginning 24 hours before the procedure) and H1 and H2 blockers (diphenhydramine, 50 mg by mouth, and cimetidine [Tagamet], 300 mg by mouth, 1 hour before the procedure).[22]

Allergic reactions to nonionic contrasts are known to exist. However, the incidence of these reactions appears to be fewer than the incidence found with the ionic media. Routine use of nonionic contrast (Isovue, Omnipaque, Optivist, Optiray) is effective and safe for facet and sacroiliac joint injections. However, when there is a chance of injection into the thecal sac (ie, epidural steroid injections), an agent that is approved for intrathecal use is recommended[23] (eg, Isovue M-200, Isovue M-300). Each contrast agent should be specifically evaluated for whether it is labeled as acceptable for intrathecal use, as some nonionic contrasts (and most ionic contrasts) are not intended for this anatomic location.

NEUROLYTIC (CYTOTOXIC) AGENTS

Neurolysis remains a relatively common procedure, but it is progressively accomplished with radiofrequency or cryogenic techniques. However, the pharmaceuticals historically used for this procedure are still useful in some locations.[1]

Chemical agents intended for neurolysis have been used for decades.[24] Commonly used agents or procedures include absolute alcohol, phenol, cryoanalgesia, and radiofrequency lesions. These materials or methods are intended to create long-term or permanent damage. This aspect must be taken into account when planning therapy and discussing the procedure with the patient.

Absolute alcohol is commercially available at 95% concentration. It causes much pain, and use at this concentration requires substantial sedation or anesthesia during injection. It is hypobaric to cerebrospinal fluid (CSF) and therefore rises if injected into the thecal sac. When injected near the sympathetic chain, alcohol destroys the ganglion cells and blocks postganglionic fibers.[25] Postinjection neuralgia, hypesthesia, and anesthesia are side effects of alcohol use.

Phenol has also been used extensively and for indications similar to that of alcohol.[26] It is a combination of carbolic acid, phenic acid, phenylic acid, phenyl hydroxide, hydroxybenzene, and oxybenzene.[27] It is not available commercially as an injectable preparation but can be made by the hospital pharmacy. It has the advantage of causing much less local pain during injection than does 95% alcohol. Phenol is usually prepared in concentrations of between 4% and 10% and is hyperbaric to CSF. It is not stable at room temperatures. Compared with alcohol, phenol produces a shorter and less-intense blockade. Moller and colleagues[28] estimated that 5% phenol was equivalent to 40% alcohol. In intractable pain, the analgesic effects of phenol and alcohol have been found to be equal.[29–33]

MATERIALS USED FOR PERCUTANEOUS VERTEBROPLASTY OR KYPHOPLASTY

Since the first procedure performed by Deramond and Galibert in 1984, polymethyl methacrylate (PMMA) has been the material of choice for percutaneous vertebroplasty (or balloon-assisted vertebroplasty, also known by the trade name of kyphoplasty). PMMA is a transparent thermoplastic that is used in many fields. Its first commercial use was as Plexiglas, which was used for the windshields and canopies of fighter airplanes in World War II. Once PMMA became available in a form that allowed on-site preparation, medical use followed, first in dental, then in joint replacement surgeries.

PMMA is composed of a liquid and powder, which are mixed together at the time of application. The active components of these materials are polymethyl methacrylate/methacrylate styrene copolymer in the powder and methyl methacrylate monomer in the liquid. Hydroquinone is added to the liquid as a stabilizer. Varying the liquid-to-powder ratios varies the setting time and mechanical behavior of the final polymer.

Methyl methacrylate is volatile, and the liquid is toxic. It was originally believed to cause the hypotension seen with bone cement implantation syndrome, but more recent research has identified fat and marrow emboli as the most likely factor.

The polymerization reaction of PMMA is exothermic and, depending on the brand and volume, may reach 100°C. The combination of temperature and monomer toxicity is the reason that a fibrous tissue layer almost always develops at the interfaces between PMMA and bone. Bone, therefore, does not bond to PMMA but rather sees it as a foreign body.

After mixing, PMMA starts out as a watery liquid and gradually and continuously increases in viscosity as it turns into a 2-dimensional, linear polymer. The material is hydrophobic. Low-, medium- and high-viscosity cements have different setting profiles and working times. In vertebroplasty, PMMA is applied in its dough-like phase.

Initially, PMMA, approved for joint surgeries or as a void filler in the skull, was used for vertebroplasty. PMMA is radiolucent, and different radiopacifying agents, such as barium sulfate, tungsten, tantalum powder, or zirconium oxide, were added at the time of mixing to allow visualization during injection using fluoroscopy.

The strength and endurance of different brands of PMMA varies due to individual composition of the liquid and powder components. A given brand of PMMA can also vary based on differences in the method of preparation. The mechanical properties depend on the powder-to-liquid ratio, the copolymer used, the particle size and quantity of radiopaque fillers, the mixing method (which influences porosity), environmental temperature, and the actual handling during the procedure. The values reported vary also according to the test method, although today there is more uniformity through the application of International Organization for Standardization (ISO) and American Society for Testing and Materials (ASTM) proscribed methods.

The mechanical test data show that PMMA is less strong and more elastic than bone and that it deforms under constant loading. As the material can help to absorb shocks, these characteristics are thought to be beneficial when used to anchor prosthetic implants. Whether PMMA is really suitable for vertebroplasty is still open to question.

Although the physical and chemical properties of PMMA are not ideal, alternatives have been slow to emerge. Instead, the focus has been on introducing more viscous variations of PMMA and on developing different pressurized delivery tools that allow the thicker cement paste to be delivered. Brand names of cements marketed for vertebroplasty include Spineplex, Vertebroplastic, Parallax, Ava-Tex, Confidence, StabiliT, BonOs, Cobalt, Opacity, Versabond, KyphX, and Vertefix.

The mechanical characteristics of different materials used in vertebroplasty are listed in Table 3.

One group of materials that have been tried as an alternative to PMMA is the resorbable self-setting cements based on calcium salts (hydroxyapatite).

Table 3
Mechanical characteristics of different materials used in vertebroplasty

Test[a]	PMMA	Calcium Salt Cements	Cortoss	Cortical Bone	ISO 5833
Compressive Strength (MPa)	73–114	5–85	200	167–215	>70
Compressive Modulus (MPa)	$1.9–3.7 \times 10^3$	—	8.0×10^3	$14.7–19.7 \times 10^3$	>1800
Compressive Fatigue (cycles to failure @ 60 MPa)	2.5×10^3	—	$>8.5 \times 10^6$	—	NA
Tensile Strength (MPa)	24–49	2–10	62	66–140	NA
Tensile Modulus (MPa)	$1.6–4.2 \times 10^3$	—	10.5×10^3	$10.9–14.8 \times 10^3$	NA
Bending Strength (MPa)	50–125	6	87	180	>50
Bending Modulus (MPa)	$1.3–2.9 \times 10^3$	—	9.7×10^3	—	NA
Creep Deformation (%)	20–50	—	<1	—	NA

Abbreviations: ISO, International Organization for Standardization; NA, not applicable; PMMA, polymethyl methacrylate.
[a] ISO 5833–2002 describes the attributes of acrylic cements for the fixation of orthopedic implants.

The compressive strength of these materials ranges from 5 to 85 MPa, and their ultimate strength is reached only 24 hours after preparation. Tensile strength is low at 2 to 10 MPa, and resistance against sheer forces is equally low. Although some good results have been reported, direct comparisons with PMMA show a higher incidence of application issues and mechanical failure for the calcium-based cements. In addition, clinical use of one of the calcium phosphate cements led to several cases of severe hypotension and death. An animal experiment showed that this result was likely because of the thrombogenic effect of the material once it leaked into the vascular system. The thrombogenicity probably varies between the different preparations, but is a concern. Today, calcium salt cements are not commonly used in vertebroplasties. Brand names of cements incorporating calcium salts include α-BSM, MIIG, Norian, BoneSource, Calcibon, Cerament, and Chronos.

In June 2009, the Food and Drug Administration (FDA) cleared a new polymer-based material for use in vertebroplasty, named Cortoss (Orthovita, Malvern, PA, USA). It consists of 3 different dimethacrylates combined with radiopaque and bioactive glass fillers. After polymerization, the resulting composite consists of a stable particle-reinforced 3-dimensionally interconnected structure. Compared with PMMA, Cortoss displays a constant, toothpaste-like viscosity, is hydrophilic, has a shorter and lower exothermic reaction (<55°C), and does not release volatile monomer during its preparation. The combination of the low exothermic reaction and the absence of volatile monomer and bioactive glass particles creates the conditions necessary for an intimate bony apposition to develop on the surface, leading to a physicochemical bonding to the host bone.

In mechanical testing, the compressive, tensile, and bending strengths were 200, 62, and 87 MPa, respectively, and the compressive, tensile, and flexural moduli were 8000; 10,500; and 9700 MPa, respectively. The mechanical characteristics of Cortoss thus are quite close to those of bone (an improvement over PMMA or hydroxyapatite).

Clinical data from a 24-month Investigational Device Exemption study submitted to the FDA directly compare Cortoss to PMMA (Spineplex). It was found that on an average, vertebroplasty with PMMA required 50% more material than with Cortoss because of a clear difference in flow and distribution patterns. Regarding all endpoints at all follow-up times, Cortoss performed at least equivalent to PMMA. It was noted that a statistically significantly higher percentage of patients who used Cortoss had successful pain relief at 3 months and function at 24 months compared with patients who used PMMA. In addition, over the 24 months duration of the study, fewer Cortoss patients experienced subsequent fractures than did PMMA patients. This difference was especially apparent in the group of patients who presented with 1 single acute fracture and no previous fractures in their history, that is, 17.6% for Cortoss versus 27.3% for PMMA. As all other parameters were equivalent between the groups, a possible relationship between fill patterns, clinical outcomes, and subsequent fracture rates will be explored further by the manufacturer.

REFERENCES

1. Mathis JM. Materials used in image-guided spine interventions. In: Mathis JM, editor. Image-guided spine interventions. New York: Springer; 2004. p. 27–36.
2. Bodduk B, Cherry D. Epidural corticosteroid agents for sciatica. Med J Aust 1985;143:402–6.
3. Dilke TF, Burry HC, Grahame R. Extradural corticosteroid injection in management of lumbar nerve root compression. Br Med J 1973;2:635–7.
4. National Health and Medical Research Council. Epidural use of steroids in the management of back pain. Canberra: Commonwealth of Australia; 1994.
5. Cicala RS, Turner R, Moran E, et al. Methylprednisolone acetate does not cause inflammatory changes in the epidural space. Anesthesiology 1990;72:556–8.
6. Delaney TJ, Rowlingson JC, Carron H, et al. Epidural steroids effects on nerves and meninges. Anesth Analg 1980;58:610–4.
7. Abram SE. Epidural steroid injections for the treatment of lumbosacral radiculopathy. J Back Musculoskeletal Rehabil 1997;8:135–49.
8. Derby R, Lee SH, Date ES, et al. Size and aggregation of corticosteroids used for epidural injections. Pain Med 2007;9(2):227–34.
9. De Jong RH. Local anesthetics, 2. St. Louis (MO): CV Mosby; 1994.
10. Eggleston ST, Lush LW. Understanding allergic reactions to local anesthetics. Ann Pharmacother 1996;30(7):851–7.
11. Clarkson CW, Hondeghern LM. Mechanism for bupivacaine depression of cardiac conduction: fast block of sodium channels during the action potential with slow recovery from block during diastole. Anesthesiology 1985;62:396–405.
12. Lee A, Fagan D, Lamont M, et al. Disposition kinetics of ropivacaine in humans. Anesth Analg 1989;69:736–8.

13. Rayburn W, Varner M, Galask R, et al. Comparison of moxalactam and cefazolin as prophylactic antibiotics during cesarean section. Antimocrob Agents Chemother 1985;27(3):337–9.

14. Boswell MV, Wolfe JR. Intrathecal cefazolin-induced seizures following attempted discography. Pain Physician 2004;7:103–6.

15. Dahl JB, Kehlet H. The value of pre-emptive analgesia in the treatment of postoperative pain. Br J Anaesth 1993;70:434–9.

16. Day R, Morrison B, Luza A, et al. A randomized trial of the efficacy and tolerability of the COX-2 inhibitor rofecoxib vs ibuprofen in patients with osteoarthiritis. Arch Intern Med 2000;160:1781–7.

17. Patt RB. Pain management. In: Abram SE, Haddox DJ, editors. The pain clinic manual. 2nd edition. Philadelphia: Lippincott Williams and Wilkins; 2000. p. 293–351.

18. Kong VK, Irwin MG. Adjuvant analgesics in neuropathic pain. Eur J Anaesthesiol 2009;26(2):96–100.

19. Freysoldt A, Fleckenstein J, Lang P, et al. Low concentrations of anitriptyline inhibit nicotinic receptors in unmyelinated axons of human peripheral nerve. Br J Pharmacol 2009;27:133–6.

20. Chiechio S, Zammataro M, Caraci F, et al. Pregabalin in the treatment of chronic pain, an overview. Clin Drug Investig 2009;29(3):203–13.

21. Safriel Y, Ang R, Ali M. Gadolinium use in spine pain management procedures for patients with contrast allergies: results in 527 patients. Cardiovasc Intervent Radiol 2008;31(2):325–31.

22. Pittman A, Castro M. Allergy and immunology. In: Ahya SN, Flood K, Paranjothi S, editors. Washington manual of medical therapeutics. 30th edition. Philadelphia: Lippincott Williams and Wilkins; 2001. p. 241–55.

23. Gries H. Chemistry of x-ray contrast agents. In: Dawson, Cosgrove, Grainger, editors. Textbook of contrast media. New York (NY): Isis Medical Media; 1999. p. 15–22.

24. Swetlow GI. Paravertebral alcohol block in cardiac pain. Am Heart J 1926;1:393.

25. Merrick RL. Degeneration and recovery of autonomic neurons following alcohol block. Ann Surg 1941;113:298.

26. Putman TJ, Hampton OJ. A technique of injection into the gasserian ganglion under roentgenographic control. Arch Neurol Psychiatry 1936;35:92–8.

27. Rathmell JP, Nelson GJ. Pharmacology of agents used during image-guided injections. In: Rathmell JP, editor. Atlas of image-guided intervention in regional anesthesia and pain medicine. Philadelphia (PA): Lippincott; 2006. p. 23–30. Chapter 4.

28. Moller JE, Helweg J, Jacobson E. Histopathological lesions in the sciatic nerve of the rat following perineural application of phenol and alcohol solutions. Dan Med Bull 1969;16:116–9.

29. Wood KA. The use of phenol as a neurolytic agent: a review. Pain 1978;5:205–29.

30. Mathis JM, Belkoff SM. Evaluation of PMMA cements altered for use in vertebroplasty. 10th Interdisciplinary Research Conference on Injectable Biomaterials. Amiens, France, March 14–15, 2000.

31. Belkoff SM, Mathis JM. In vitro biomechanical evaluation of bone cements used in percutaneous vertebroplasty. Bone 1999;25:23S–5S.

32. Jasper LE, Deramond H, Mathis JM. The effects of monomer-to-powder ratio on the material properties of Cranioplastic. Bone 1999;25:27S–9S.

33. Tohmeh AG, Mathis SM, Belkoff SM. Biomechanical efficacy of unipedicular versus bipedicular vertebroplasty for the management of osteoporotic compression fractures. Spine 1999;24:1772–6.

Percutaneous Lumbar Discectomy

Stanley Golovac, MD

KEYWORDS

- Percutaneous lumbar discectomy • Discogenic pain
- Annulus • Annular breakdown and tears
- Intervertebral disc
- Percutaneous needle insertion and placement
- Alternative to open discectomy

Estimated to cost the United States health care system more than $20 billion a year,[1,2] discogenic leg pain represents the primary cause of health care expenditure. Taken together, back pain and discogenic leg pain result in more days lost than any other combined illnesses and injuries.

Annular breakdown and tears are common discogenic sources that produce pain,[3,4] and are usually treated with microdiscectomy by orthopedic surgeons and neurosurgeons. Open discectomy has been considered to be the gold standard for relieving pressure on nerve roots. By decompressing the nerve root from the disc, neurologic function is usually restored and pain is relieved. Recurrent disc herniations may and typically do occur[5] because of the annular violation that results from the surgical procedure.

Many percutaneous procedures that specifically focus on disc herniation have been developed over the last several decades. These procedures have included chemonucleolysis, automated/manual percutaneous nucleotomy, laser treatments, intradiscal thermal annuloplasty and, more recently, nucleoplasty and Dekompressor. All these procedures are designed to reduce intradiscal pressure, so that the protruded disc area can retract back into place, given that there is enough elastogenicity to allow recovery.

ANATOMY

A central cartilaginous fibrous ring having sensitive nerve endings surrounding the outer rim anatomically comprises the intervertebral disc.[6] The nucleus is bordered superiorly and inferiorly by dense cartilage and bony endplates from the respective vertebral surfaces (Fig. 1).

Composed of an inner and outer layer, the annulus is loosely attached to the anterior longitudinal ligament and is strongly attached to the posterior longitudinal ligament. This structure explains why axial back pain results when a central-disc protrusion occurs. The pain occurs when the fibers pull away from their attachments because of the ligamentous displacement from the annulus and the vertebral body. The nucleus, a notochordal remnant that is relatively avascular in the adult and is not significantly innervated, acts as a cushion. The annulus is a highly innervated structure in which the sinu-vertebral nerve wraps around the posterior aspect. Substance P and unmyelinated C fibers have been shown to be present in the annulus (Fig. 2).

The intervertebral disc functions to provide a surface area to distribute stress absorption and motion restriction.[2] The annulus serves to contain the nuclear material and to restrict longitudinal and rotational motion between spinal segments. Fibers in the annulus are arranged in variable directions in each fibrous layer to provide support in multiple directions. Approximately 20 of these are arranged anteriorly and 12 to 15 are arranged posteriorly.

INTERVERTEBRAL DISCS IN SPINAL PAIN

It is thought that discogenic pain originates from the sinu-vertebral nerves that innervate the outer annulus of the discs. Discogenic pain is provoked

Disclosures: Consultant for Stryker Corporation and St. Jude Medical Neuro Division.
Space Coast Pain Institute, 595 North Courtenay Parkway, Merritt Island, Florida 32953, USA
E-mail address: sgolovac@mac.com

Neuroimag Clin N Am 20 (2010) 223–227
doi:10.1016/j.nic.2010.02.009

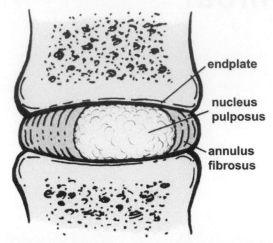

Fig. 1. Sagittal diagram showing the anatomy of the lumbar intervertebral disc. The soft inner nucleus pulposus is encircled by the fibrous bands of the annulus, which are thinner posteriorly. (*Reprinted from* Mathis JM, editor. Image-guided spine interventions. New York: Springer Science + Business Media; 2004; with permission.)

by any factor that produces an inflammatory response from the chemical mediators in the disc. Phospholipase A and prostaglandins are known irritants to the outer nerve supply and thereby produce pain and inflammation. Typically seen when axial loading results in pain during standing and extending the spine, discogenic pain is described as stabbing, knifelike, or burning in nature.

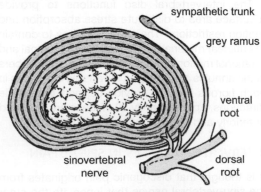

Fig. 2. Axial cross section showing the innervation of the intervertebral disc. Although there is no significant innervation of the nucleus, the annulus is innervated with unmyelinated fibers, primarily by way of the sinu-vertebral nerve. Pain fibers are present throughout the disc but most densely in the posterior annulus. (*Reprinted from* Mathis JM, editor. Image-guided spine interventions. New York: Springer Science + Business Media; 2004; with permission.)

There are many theories about the exact patho-physiology of the pain mechanism, but most revolve around pathologic tears of the posterior annulus of the disc and mechanical or chemical stimulation of nociceptive receptors, located in and around the posterior annulus fibrosus, relayed through the sinu-vertebral nerve.

Present therapy, which has remained unchanged for many years, includes rest, relaxation, anti-inflammatory agents, and application of ice to the affected areas. Limited exercise, stretching, and aquatic body posturing are then introduced. If the pain does not improve with conservative measures, interventional therapies such as trigger injections, nerve conduction blockade, and central nervous system blocks (ie, epidural steroids, radiofrequency ablation, and sympathetic blockade) may have a place in the course of treatment.

If surgical intervention is needed to restore normal nerve function, it should only be considered when a neurologic deficit causes loss of reflexes, sensory deficits, or weakness. This surgical intervention may be a minimally invasive microdiscectomy, laminectomy, or foraminotomy or an extensive fusion. Other considerations include morbidity, cost, loss of work time, rehabilitation, the possibility of developing chronic pain, and medication dependency.

HISTORICAL PERSPECTIVE

In the 1990s, percutaneous procedures were developed as a minimally invasive treatment to relieve discogenic and radicular pain, and to reduce morbidity. Gary Onik,[7] an interventional radiologist, initiated percutaneous needle insertion; he believed that by introducing a trocar into the nucleus, it was possible to extract disc material and reduce the outer bulges that compressed or irritated nerve roots. In 2000, the Saal brothers invented the intradiscal electrothermy procedure that involved placing a heating element into the posterior nuclear annulus interface; the regelatinization of the proteoglycan fibers sealed off the annular tears. Several studies have shown an improvement of 40%.[8]

In 2000, ArthroCare Spine introduced the Nucleoplasty (ArthoCare Corporation, Austin, TX, USA) wand that allows a practitioner to create channels in the disc. These channels create voids in which disc bulge can retract. Whether the radiofrequency energy or physical change in the disc reduces overall pain remains to be proven. In 2002, Stryker Corporation introduced the Dekompressor (Stryker Corporation, Kalamazoo, MI, USA) device (**Fig. 3**) to percutaneously remove

DEKOPRESSOR

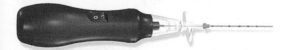

Fig. 3. Dekompressor device. (*Courtesy of* Stryker Corporation, Kalamazoo, MI, USA; with permission.)

disc material. This device yields a specimen for quantitative and qualitative analysis, and provides proof of what and how much was removed.[9,10]

INDICATIONS AND PROCEDURE: NEEDLE PLACEMENT

Inclusion and exclusion criteria are very important for the desired outcome. Magnetic resonance imaging findings must be verified first with an anteroposterior (AP) view and then with a lateral view (**Fig. 4**). Before proceeding with a percutaneous discectomy, pain relief should be confirmed after a selective nerve root block has been performed.

Bulged Disc

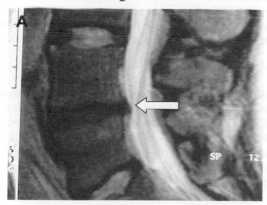

Axial view

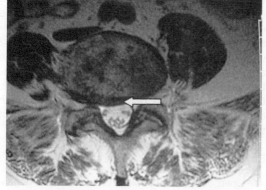

Fig. 4. (*A*) Contained bulged disc at lumbar vertebra L4. (*B*) Axial view of right-paravertebral disc bulge.

To begin the procedure, place the patient in a prone position. Minimal sedation can be induced by titrating drugs such as midazolam (Versed [Hoffmann-LaRoche Inc, Nutley, NJ, USA]) and fentanyl, to reduce anxiety and help control blood pressure-related changes. The targeted area must be cleansed and sterilized with povidone-iodine (Betadine) and alcohol preparation. Position the fluoroscope to view the spine in an AP view, and align the endplates and pedicles. Next, one should rotate the scope by approximately 30° to an oblique position or until the superior articulating process (SAP) bisects the endplates. Once the disc is clearly seen lateral to the SAP, the objective target is in sight.

Anesthetize the skin and deeper fascial plane by using a 3.5-in spinal needle to further place local anesthetic solution toward the SAP. Introduce the 17-gauge Crawford needle into the outer annulus and puncture the disc; the needle should enter the disc and stay in the posterior aspect of the disc itself. The first view should be an AP view that allows visualization of the needle's entrance to determine whether it has crossed the midline mark.

The best way to ensure optimal position of the needle is to visualize the pedicle and spinous process. Drawing a line between the 2 allows for a clear reference that the needle tip is in the middle of the disc (**Fig. 5**). This alignment is visualized in a lateral view that illustrates the needle tip in the posterior one-third of the vertebral body. The image will indicate that the distal tip of auger will be located in the nuclear-annular junction. On an

P-P line

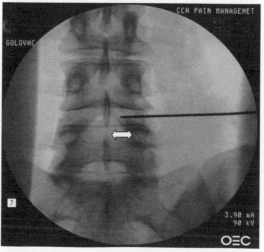

Fig. 5. P-P line. Proper needle placement midway between the spinous process and pedicle denoting correct placement of the introducer needle.

AP view, the needle tip should not pass beyond the spinous process (**Fig. 6**).

Next, turn on the Dekompressor and slightly push the unit in and out approximately 1 cm (**Fig. 7**). After running the device for 2 minutes, remove the probe, cut off its distal portion, and send it to pathology for quantitative and qualitative analysis. Clean the lower back area with alcohol. Apply Neosporin (Johnson & Johnson, New Brunswick, NJ, USA) ointment over the puncture site and use a bandage to cover the needle site.

The patient is then transferred to a preparatory and discharge area, and can be discharged after an uneventful recovery with instructions to not bend, twist, flex, or squat for the next 24 hours. Physical therapy should follow as an integral part of rehabilitation, and should focus on

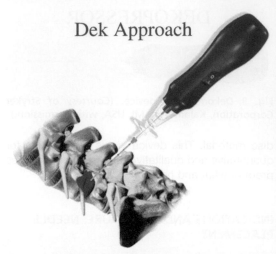

Fig. 7. Dekompressor device in oblique view noted to enter the affected side. (*Courtesy of* Stryker Corporation, Kalamazoo, MI; with permission.)

aqua exercises and dynamic progressive strengthening.

After 4 weeks of continued rehabilitation, the patient should be reevaluated to determine his or her level of improvement. If pain and radicular symptoms are not improved to the physician's satisfaction, a surgical consult can be requested to determine surgical candidacy.

COMPLICATIONS AND CONSENT

All procedures may produce complications that must be considered before the procedure. Complications include infection, bleeding, nerve root injury, disc infection (discitis), blood vessel injury, and the remote chance of death. All complications should be covered in the risks, alternatives, and benefits sections of the consent form.

SUMMARY

When strict criteria are followed, the expected outcome is measured at approximately 75%. The evaluation period includes postprocedural rehabilitation of 2 weeks of aqua therapy and then 2 weeks of progressive functional exercises. At the completion of 4 weeks of rehabilitation, a reevaluation is performed, and the definitive outcome is then measured. If a persistent mechanical pain exists, either a discogram or selective nerve root sleeve should be performed.

REFERENCES

1. Lipetz JS. Pathophysiology of inflammatory, degenerative and cooperative radiculopathies. Phys Med Rehabil Clin N Am 2002;13:439–49.

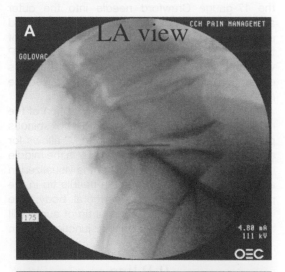

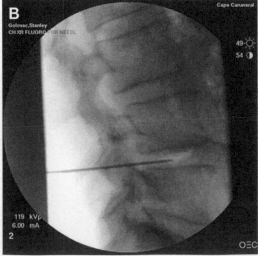

Fig. 6. (*A, B*) Lateral view of needle placement showing the introducer in the posterior one-third of the vertebral body.

2. Carey TS, Garrett J, Jackman A, et al. The outcomes and costs of care for acute low back pain among patients seen by primary care practitioners, chiropractors, and orthopedic surgeons. The North Carolina back pain project. N Engl J Med 1995;333:913–7.
3. Prescher A. Anatomy and pathophysiology of the aging spine. Eur J Radiol 1998;27:181–95.
4. Coppers MH, Marani E, Thomeer RT, et al. Innervation of painful lumbar discs. Spine (Phila Pa 1976) 1997;22:2342–50.
5. Carragee EJ, Hahn M, Suen P, et al. Clinical outcomes after lumbar discectomy for sciatica: the effects of fragment type and anular competence. J Bone Joint Surg Am 2003;85-A:102–8.
6. Haines SJ, Jordan N, Boen JR, et al. Discectomy strategies for lumbar disc herniations: results of the LAPDOG trial. J Clin Neurosci 2002;9(4): 411–7.
7. Onik GM, Helms CA, Ginsberg L, et al. Percutaneous lumbar discectomy using a new aspiration probe. AJR Am J Roentgenol 1985;6:290–3.
8. Saal JS, Saal JA. Management of chronic discogenic low back pain with a thermal intradiscal catheter. A preliminary report. Spine (Phila Pa 1976) 2000; 25(3):382–8.
9. Alo KM, Wright RE, Sutcliffe J, et al. Percutaneous lumbar discectomy. Clinical response in an initial cohort of fifty consecutive patients with chronic radicular pain. Pain Pract 2004;4(1):19–29.
10. Amoretti N, David P, Gimaud A, et al. Clinical follow-up of 50 patients treated by percutaneous lumbar discectomy. Clin Imaging 2006;30:242–4.

Minimally Invasive Dynamic Stabilization of the Degenerated Lumbar Spine

Giuseppe Bonaldi, MD

KEYWORDS

- Dynamic stabilization • Spine stabilization
- Spine biomechanics • Minimally invasive spine surgery
- Motion preservation

The skull essentially protects the brain. The spine, made of a series of joints, has motion as its primary function, at the same time protecting the spinal cord. The basic spinal functional unit (SU) is the smallest physiologic motion unit of the spine and therefore is termed, *a motion segment*. It consists of 2 adjacent vertebrae, the disc, and all the connecting ligaments. Individual motion segments contribute to the total motion of the spine. Abnormal motion in an SU is defined as vertebral or spinal instability. Myriad biomechanical, clinical, and radiologic definitions of spinal instability are available.[1–3] The definition by the American Academy of Orthopaedic Surgeons states, "Segmental instability is an abnormal response to applied loads, characterized by motion in motion segments beyond normal constraints." Motion in degenerated joints (ie, beyond the normal limits of the joint itself) generates pain. Eliminating motion in an abnormal SU seems to eliminate pain. Most orthopedic surgery for the degenerated lumbar spine, entailing various fusion (ie, locking of 2 or more vertebrae as a single unit) techniques, with or without instrumentation, is based on this principle. Disadvantages and problems of traditional fusion methods are loss of mobility and curvature, altered sagittal balance, instrumentation failure, harvest site pain, infection, and transference of load (stress) to adjacent levels. Such surgery, moreover, is not easily reversible. The main concern of fusion surgery is the impact on the adjacent levels, in particular facet joints

and discs, structures that are then overloaded. After fusion surgery, these may consequently deteriorate (**Fig. 1**).[4–8] Hilibrand and colleagues[9] have estimated that after cervical fusion there is 25% symptomatic adjacent level disease at 10 years; Ghiselli and colleagues[10] estimate 36% at 10 years after lumbar fusion.

All of these issues have led to attempts to develop new motion preservation technologies for surgical treatment of spinal instability, commonly referred to as dynamic stabilization. Dynamic stabilization has been defined as "a system that would alter favorably the movement and load transmission of a spinal motion segment, without the intention of fusion of the segment."[11] Dynamic stabilization tries to introduce a more gradual, intermediate therapeutic step between abnormal movement of the SUs (instability) and total absence of movement (fusion). The most significant advances in this field were made in the past 10 to 15 years; during the same period a gradual shift toward a minimally invasive approach of spinal surgery was technically developed and accepted. During this period, attention of biomechanics experts and spine surgeons was mainly focused on the posterior structures of the spine, facets, and spinous processes, for 2 reasons: these structures are easily accessible by a minimally invasive approach and an action on them determined by different devices can largely modify the functional behavior of the SU. The combination of 2 concepts, preservation of

Department of Neuroradiology, Riuniti Hospital, Largo Barozzi 1. 24128 Bergamo, Italy
E-mail address: mail@bonaldi.org

Neuroimag Clin N Am 20 (2010) 229–241
doi:10.1016/j.nic.2010.02.010
1052-5149/10/$ – see front matter © 2010 Elsevier Inc. All rights reserved.

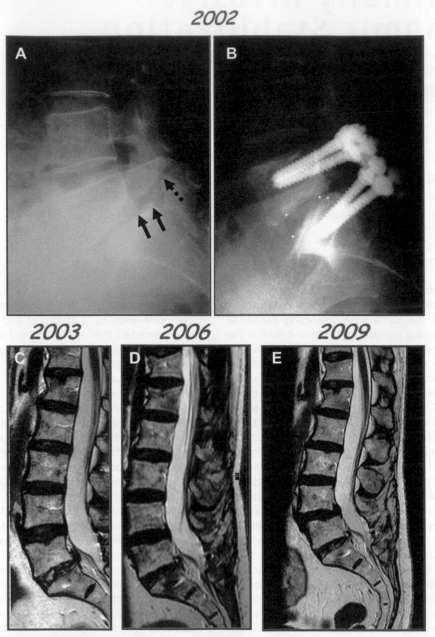

Fig. 1. (*A*) L5-S1 spondilolisthesis (*arrows*) due to bilateral isthmic lysis (*dotted arrow*), surgically treated in 2002 by instrumented rigid fusion (*B*). (*C–E*) The modification of dynamic loads carries in few years to a degenerative, no lytic spondilolisthesis of the adjacent L4-L5 level.

motion and minimal surgical invasiveness, seems to be opening a new era in surgery for the degenerated spine. The radiologic community, which has always been in the forefront of developing and performing minimally invasive interventions for the degenerated spine (percutaneous discectomies, vertebroplasty, and other procedures) is well situated to participate in applying these innovations.

BASIC BIOMECHANICS

The SU is extremely complex in its components and movements. Thus, there can be many different sources of pain in pathologic situations. Unfortunately, the biomechanics of SUs are neither fully understood nor simple to explain. This article summarizes the main concepts on which the designs of the different devices are

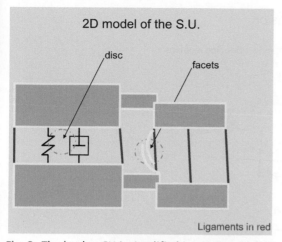

2D model of the S.U.

disc

facets

Ligaments in red

Fig. 2. The lumbar SU is simplified in a 2-D model, in which torque and lateral bending movements are eliminated. Such movements are not or only partially affected by the dynamic stabilization devices.

based, simplifying the 3-D anatomy and physiology of the SU to a 2-D model (**Fig. 2**) (ie, essentially eliminating the torque and lateral bending movements, which are not, or almost not, affected by the dynamic devices).

In flexion and extension, muscles apply a bending moment to the SU. A bending moment (M) corresponds to 2 vector forces applied in opposite directions with a distance between them different from 0 and is measured as a force (F) multiplied by a distance (d): M = Fd (**Fig. 3**). During flexion of the lumbar spine, muscles apply a bending moment to the SUs (**Fig. 4**).

The total motion obtained (modification of posture from neutral to flexion) is the sum of the modifications obtained at the level of every single SU (ie, a decrease of the anterior disc height [$\Delta z2$] and a widening [defined by the angle between the spinous processes: $\alpha\Delta$] of the

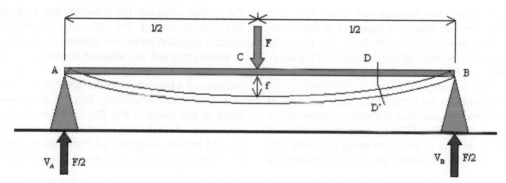

Fig. 3. A bending moment exists in a structural element when a moment is applied to the element so that the element bends. Moments and torques are measured as a force multiplied by a distance: M = Fd.

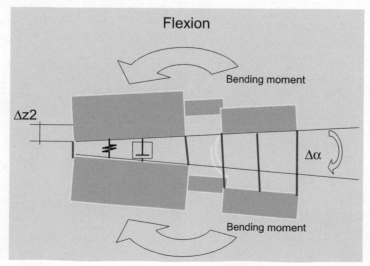

Flexion

Bending moment

$\Delta z2$

$\Delta\alpha$

Bending moment

Fig. 4. The bending moment applied by muscles in flexion to the SU determines an asymmetric decrease of the height of the disc and an opening of the posterior bony elements.

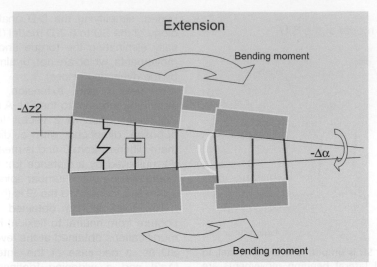

Fig. 5. In extension, the bending moment determines an asymmetric increase of the height of the disc, whereas the posterior bony elements get closer, with the angle determined by the 2 spinous processes becoming negative.

posterior structures, which are stretched and opened). The supraspinous ligament is the structure limiting flexion more effectively. The opposite happens in extension, with an increase in the anterior disc height and closing of the interspinous space, with the angle becoming negative (**Fig. 5**). Two concepts to be acquainted with are that of neutral zone (NZ) and that of instantaneous center of rotation (ICR). The NZ (**Fig. 6**) is the position of the SU in which a small bending moment can obtain a large movement (ie, a large change of

the angles between the 2 vertebrae). In a normal SU, the center of the NZ corresponds to the middle position between flexion and extension; a small moment is required to start flexion (or extension), but with progressive increase of the movement it becomes harder and harder to obtain new flexion (or extension). The NZ is a measurement of the laxity of the SU, and it widens in the presence of instability. Pathologic widening of the NZ allows exaggerated movements, which in turn require a large amount of energy for return

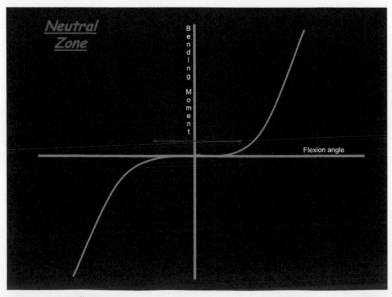

Fig. 6. Bending moment versus flexion angle of a SU. In the NZ, small differences in bending moment result in large changes of angle.

to the neutral state. Dynamic devices aim to reduce the NZ or to reposition it in the proper (not painful) place.

The ICR corresponds to the point at which, if a load is applied, no bending occurs. It is defined as instantaneous, because it can change at every instant, during different types of movements. As an example, think of a bike's wheel. When the wheel turns around the central pivot not touching the ground, the ICR corresponds to the not moving center of the hub, but in a running bike the only not moving part is the one touching the ground, and it changes at every instant (imagine the wheel turning as a whole around the fixed point in contact with the ground). It is difficult to predict the ICR in structures as complex as the SU. It changes with different movements, and these changes become more unpredictable in the presence of instability. More often, in a healthy SU in the standing, inactive position, the ICR is located posterior to the center of the disc, just above the inferior end plate[12] (approximately corresponding to the center of gravity). It moves in flexion-extension, and the variability is considerable. There are no simple rules to predict the effect of stabilization devices on the ICR, but one is notable: the ICR moves toward an increase of stiffness. What happens when an interspinous spacer is deployed? Things are not modified in flexion (if the supraspinous process is surgically preserved); in extension, the movement is not modified until the spacer goes under compression.

At that moment (Fig. 7), if the spacer is rigid and provided that the bone does not fail (break) (see Fig. 7 for the weakest points of the posterior arch, which are possible sites of failure), an additional increase in the anterior height of the disc is obtained ($-\Delta z3$), with stretching of the anterior annulus. To allow and compensate for this, the facets move opposite to the normal direction, opening instead of closing. In other words, the movement, which is no longer obtainable at the expense of the interspinous space (decrease of the angle in extension [see Fig. 5]) is now obtained at the level of different, elastic structures. An immediate consequence is that back pain induced in extension by pressure originating in the facets or posterior annulus of the lumbar spine may be relieved by unloading of facets or posterior annulus generated by the interspinous decompression.[13] In a similar way, is it possible to unload the whole disc, when it is surmised as the source of pain? The disc is extremely stiff, and only minimal increase-decrease in disc height can be obtained under axial compression-distraction ($\Delta z1$ in Fig. 8). The disc can be unloaded only if the load is transferred to a device/instrumentation, but implants are not stiff enough to accomplish that task. For this reason, stand-alone instrumented fusions fail in the long term if bony fusion does not take place. This is a general rule of fusion surgery: a fusion cannot be expected to be obtained simply by hardware, because the action of the hardware is temporary. Its action is to allow for actual bone fusion to take place. Otherwise, instrumentation (even metallic ones) and contact surfaces with bone fail in the mid or long term. The disc, however, is compliant in flexion-

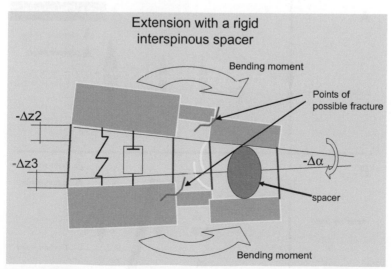

Fig. 7. Extension with a rigid interspinous spacer. An additional increase in disc height is obtained, while the facets move opposite to normal, opening instead of closing. The weakest bony structures are indicated by the light brown lines (*arrows*).

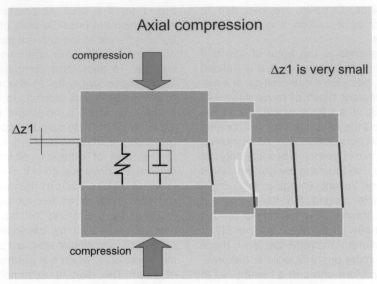

Fig. 8. Axial compression of a SU. Only a small decrease in disc height is obtained.

extension, because of posterior and anterior shifting of the nucleus pulposus in flexion-extension. Thus, if posterior stabilization devices cannot have a primary role in unloading the disc, they can have a profound effect on the loads of specific regions of the disc. Fig. 9 depicts the effects of a tension band (tying the upper and lower spinous processes to the interspinous device), which give an additional moment to resist bending. In a normal/uninstrumented condition, the ICR in flexion moves anteriorly, whereas the action of the tension bend keeps it more posterior, limiting

its shifting. The consequence is a reduction of compression forces on the anterior annulus and reduction of tension on posterior annulus and facets. Alternatively (Fig. 10), the rigid interspinous spacer in extension moves the ICR posteriorly behind the facets (ie, toward the increase of stiffness determined by the device), modifying the loads on the different parts of the SU: the load on facets and posterior annulus is reduced instead of increased (tension instead of usual compression). Thus, with wise use of the correct device, the loads can be moved away from painful areas,

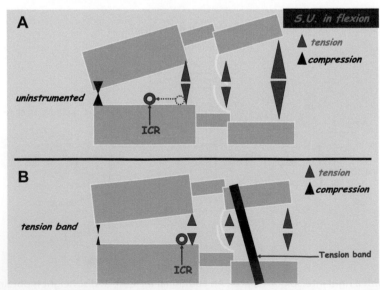

Fig. 9. A tension band gives an additional moment resisting bending, thus reducing compression on the anterior annulus and tension on posterior annulus and facets.

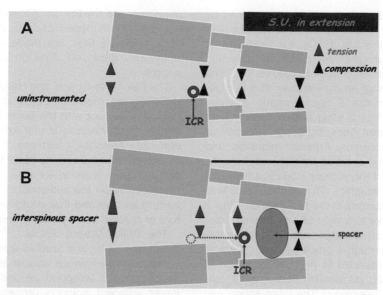

Fig. 10. The rigid interspinous spacer moves the ICR posteriorly, modifying the loads on the different parts of the SU (see text).

giving relief to patients and at the same time preserving motion in the SUs.

DESIGN RATIONALE OF DIFFERENT DEVICES AND GENERAL SURGICAL PRINCIPLES

Regarding dynamic stabilization devices, the only surgical approaches to date that can be considered minimally invasive, and widely available to clinical practice, are the posterior ones, for anatomic reasons. Anterior approaches for nonfusion procedures, such as the ones for total disc replacements (prostheses), still require open procedures. Nucleus replacements (replacing the nucleus only, with the advantage of cartilage and annulus preservation) are under ongoing development and evaluation. Many different materials are proposed, the most promising among them represented by injectable polymers. No single system is

widely available in clinical practice or truly minimally invasive.

Posterior stabilization devices fall into 2 main categories of design: interspinous spacers (with or without tension bands) and pedicle screw-based systems. The bands are passed around the upper and lower spinous processes and then tied to the interspinous component, with the double purpose of securing the device and (in some devices) limiting flexion/rotation. Rigid, non-deformable interspinous spacers have a constant effect on the distraction of the spinous processes, whereas low-rigidity, deformable spacers act more as shock absorbers, with a consequent, more physiologic action on range of motion of the SU together with an increase of bone compliance.

The interspinous process decompression system X-STOP (**Fig. 11**) (St. Francis Medical

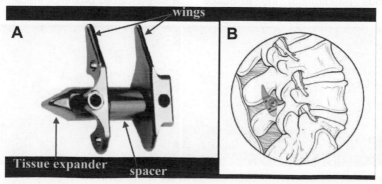

Fig. 11. (*A*) Image of the X-STOP, depicting the lateral wings, the central spacer, and the tissue expander. (*B*) The device deployed in the interspinous ligament, with the wings limiting lateral migration.

Technologies, Alameda, CA, USA, now owned by Medtronic) was proposed by Zucherman and colleagues[14] in the late 1990s, for treatment of symptoms of neurogenic intermittent claudication (INC) due to segmental spinal stenosis.[15–17] The X-STOP consists of an oval spacer that is positioned between the 2 symptomatic spinous processes. The lateral wing is then attached to prevent the implant from migrating anteriorly or laterally out of position. Anterior migration and posterior migration are also limited, respectively, by the lamina and the supraspinous ligament (the latter not being violated). The central pivot was rigid, made of titanium, in the first version. Now it is semirigid thanks to a layer of polyetheretherketone (PEEK) (discussed later) external to the metal. It is deployed through a small posterior surgical approach. It is intended to prevent extension of the stenotic levels, yet allowing flexion, axial rotation, and lateral bending.[18] The intervention can be performed under local anesthesia and mild sedation, without removing any bone or soft tissues, with preservation of the supraspinous ligament. Leaving in place and intact the supraspinous ligament has the double of effect not only preventing posterior migration of the device but also not modifying the behavior of the SU in flexion. The procedure is typically done with a 24-hour hospitalization.

Biomechanical studies have shown that the implant significantly reduces intradiscal pressure and facets load and prevents narrowing of the spinal canal and neural foramens.[13,19,20] It provides an alternative therapy to conservative treatment and decompressive surgery for patients suffering from INC, and its safety and effectiveness were confirmed in a randomized, controlled trial.[14,21,22]

There are similar devices on the European market, not yet approved in the United States (where, however, many clinical trials are ongoing), such as the Falena (Mikaï), the Superion (Verti-Flex), the Aperius (Medtronic), the In-Space (Synthes), and the BacJac (Pioneer Surgical Technology). The Superion and the Aperius are both rigid, because they are made of titanium, and both are deployed through a percutaneous approach.

The Falena, In-Space, and BacJac, similar to the X-STOP, are made of PEEK in the part of the device in contact with the bone. PEEK is a semicrystalline thermoplastic that exhibits a combination of strength, stiffness, resilience, and biocompatibility, which is ideal for use in orthopedic surgery. It allows for stress to be distributed more evenly on the surrounding bony structures, limiting an overload that could lead to acute fracture or chronic bone porosity and resorption.

The Wallis (Abbot Spine)[23–25] and the DIAM (Medtronic)[26,27] are double-action devices, in which the interspinous spacer is secured with 2 tension bands wrapped around the upper and lower adjacent spinous processes. The bands also give support to the supraspinous ligament in limiting flexion of the SU (hence the double-action of the devices, more intense for the Wallis and less for the DIAM, whose surgical insertion does not entail sectioning of the supraspinous ligament).

The spacer of the Wallis is made of PEEK. The spacer of the DIAM is made of silicone, which is more resilient and compressible, and it is preloaded by compression before insertion, thus permitting a posterior tensioning of the ligaments and disc, allowing a type of ligamentotaxis, particularly of the posterior annulus fibrosus.

Other devices, based on different concepts, that are more rigid (less dynamic in their action) are the Coflex (Paradigm Spine), a U-shaped titanium device, surgically inserted between the spinous processes, and the Aspen (Lanx Laboratories), available in the United States since January 2008, which helps promote fusion to achieve a solid construct through an interspinous arthrodesis.

The PercuDyn (Interventional Spine) (Fig. 12) is a screw-based posterior stabilization device. Two

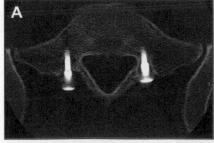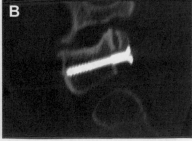

Fig. 12. The screw-based PercuDyn system: titanium screws are anchored in the S1 pedicles (A), whereas the polycarbonate-urethane heads of the screws support and cushion the inferior facet complex of the upper metamer (B), limiting its extension and unloading the disc.

screws are anchored, with a totally percutaneous, fluoroscopy-guided approach, through the pedicles into the vertebral body, so that the polycarbonate-urethane resilient heads provide support to the inferior articular facets (of the upper vertebra), limiting their range of motion in extension. The device can be used in anatomic situations where a spinous process is not present (L5-S1 or postlaminectomy). Moreover, the device might have a more efficient ability to treat discogenic pain. The spacer is mounted more anteriorly with respect to a true interspinous device. Consequently, it exerts a more efficient action in moving the ICR outside the disc, forcing the segment into flexion in neutral position and keeping the posterior annulus as distracted as possible. Thus, on a theoretic, biomechanical basis it should decrease intradiscal pressure, reduce annular compression, and preserve posterior disc height in a more efficient way than more posteriorly applied devices.[28]

PATIENT SELECTION CRITERIA

Rigid or semirigid interspinous devices, such as the X-STOP, Falena, Aperius or In-Space, were developed for treatment of symptoms of INC due to segmental spinal stenosis.[15-17] Symptoms of INC are pain and discomfort radiating to buttocks, thigh, and lower limbs during standing and walking. This is exacerbated by lumbar extension and relieved by flexion. Standing narrows the neural foramina and canal area resulting in impingement, whereas flexing (such as when sitting or riding a bike) increases the area relieving impingement. The primary level affected is L4-L5,

followed by L3-L4. In extension, the implant significantly increases the canal area by 18% (231 to 273 mm^2), the subarticular diameter by 50% (2.5 to 3.7 mm), the canal diameter by 10% (17.8 to 19.5 mm), the foraminal area by 25% (106 to 133 mm^2), and the foraminal width by 41% (3.4 to 4.8 mm).[19] The final effect is that the implant prevents narrowing of the spinal canal and foramina in extension, thus reducing or eliminating nerve root compression. In patients with symptomatic lumbar spinal stenosis who underwent MRI before and after implantation of the X-STOP, the device increased the cross-sectional area of the dural sac and exit foramina without causing changes in posture.[29] Significant increase in the dimensions of the neural foramen and canal area were also demonstrated after surgery.[30] **Fig. 13** illustrates reduction of the anterolisthesis and widening of the spinal canal after insertion of an interspinous Aperius device.

This indication for interspinous device implant was validated by a randomized, controlled, prospective, multicenter trial comparing patients treated with the X-STOP with patients treated nonoperatively. A total 191 patients were treated, 100 in the X-STOP group and 91 in the control group. The conclusions of the study are that the X-STOP provides a conservative yet effective treatment for patients suffering from lumbar spinal stenosis.[14,21,22] To date the X-STOP is the only device approved by the Food and Drug Administration for treatment of INC.

Indications for control of axial pain are less clear-cut. They remain poorly defined and largely left to a surgeon's personal opinions and

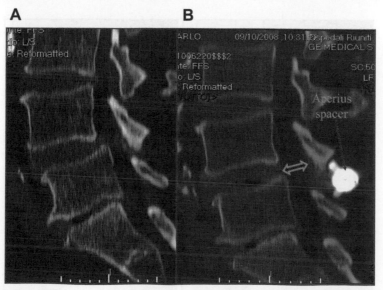

Fig. 13. The rigid, percutaneous Aperius interspinous spacer reduces the degenerative spondilolisthesis and widens the sagittal diameter of the spinal canal. (*A*) Preoperative; (*B*) postoperative.

experience. Reliable data are still lacking, but ongoing trials are studying many devices (Wallis, DIAM, In-Space, Superion, and Coflex). Most studies are focused on moderate degenerative lumbar stenosis at 1 or 2 levels or treatment of mild to moderate degenerative disc disease of the lumbar spine. The estimated study completions are projected to be from 2011 to 2013 (although enrollment is already terminated in a few cases). Hopefully they will provide the necessary evidence for appropriate choices in clinical practice.

In a study of cadavers on the effects of an interspinous implant on disc pressures, Swanson and colleagues[18] reported that the posterior annulus and nucleus pulposus pressures were reduced by 63% and 41%, respectively, during extension, and by 38% and 20%, respectively, in the neutral, standing position. The most frequent indications are early disc degeneration (the so-called "black disc", which is an incorrect, nonradiologic definition that is widely used in surgical communities), contained disc herniations, mild segmental instability (postsurgical or not), and facet syndrome (with hypertrophy, osteophytosis, cysts, and incongruity). The indications proposed by Sénégas[25] for the Wallis are significant loss of disc material after surgery, degenerative disc adjacent to a fused segment, and isolated Modic 1[31] lesion attributable to chronic low back pain. Another indication is providing a cushioning mechanism to SU adjacent to fused levels.

The principles of biomechanics (described previously) should direct surgical strategy. The rigid or semirigid interspinous component limits extension, moving the ICR and the loads away from facets and posterior annulus. The tension bands limit flexion and rotation, adding stability and helping restore the alignment of the metamers. Changes in the location of the ICR change the deformation of local areas of tissue, moving the distribution of loads. Unloading of facets was discussed previously. In a case as is illustrated in **Fig. 14**, the source of pain is presumably in the anterior inflammatory osteocondrosis, and the surgical strategy should rely more on a limitation of flexion (ie, on the posterior tension band to reduce anterior disc load). The interspinous spacer partially limits the load on the anterior disc, however, forcing the facets to open instead of closing in extension (discussed previously; see **Figs. 9** and **10**). For this reason almost all devices with a tension band are double-action devices, coupling bands and an interspinous spacer. Such systems tend to add stability to the vertebral segment, at the same time limiting the extremes of flexion and extension (ie, reducing the NZ that was widened by the pathologic conditions) and restoring a range of motion as physiologic as possible. They increase resistance to compression and stretch, not (or only partially) affecting rotation and lateral bending.

The normal annulus (**Fig. 15**) resists the pressure transmitted by the radial expansion of the nucleus, compressed during physiologic loads, with an outward bulging of its fibers in the horizontal plane, thus acting in tension rather then compression. When the nucleus degenerates, its

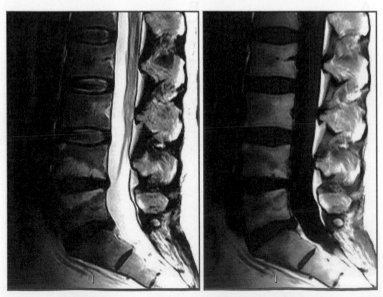

Fig. 14. Anterior, partially inflammatory (mixed Modic 1 and 2) osteocondrosis of the L4-L5 disc space.

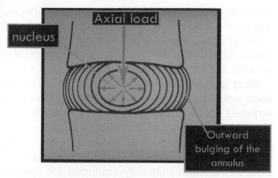

Fig. 15. Normal disc. The pressure exerted by the compressive loads on the hydrated nucleus is transmitted in a radial direction, determining an outward bulging of the fibers of the annulus in the horizontal plane.

mechanical properties change; it can no longer expand under loads and, therefore, the annular fibers are no longer forced out radially; they act in compression rather then tension and this results in annular tears, fissures, and possible painful tissue. In cases, as in **Fig. 16**, an origin of pain could be presumed from the hyperintensity zone in the posterior annulus. In early degeneration, there is sprouting of vessels, accompanied by nociceptive fibers, from the outer toward the inner disc, and this becomes painful owing to the presence of nodules of granulation tissue, sometimes evident on MRI as zones of high signal, usually in the posterior annulus.[32] In such situations, the aim is to move the load away from the posterior annulus by means of the action on the ICR of a rigid posterior

interspinous device. The action of the device could in theory reverse the wrong load condition on the annulus, favoring its regeneration and nucleus rehydration. Among the advantages of preservation of motion is that normal loads and motion are essential to maintain all joints in good health, because these conditions provide the ideal nutrition of the articular components. This is true for the intervertebral disc, which is not vascularized and consequently whose nutrition and oxygenation only come from osmotic diffusion from the surrounding tissues, particularly through permeability of the cartilage endplates. Nutrients are in a way pumped into the disc, and movement plays a major role in this mechanism. When treating discogenic pain, the degeneration of the disc must be limited to grades 1 to 4 of Pfirrmann and coworkers'[33] classification and diffused Modic changes should be excluded.

Rigid or semirigid interspinous spacers may help reduce minimal degrees of degenerative spondilolisthesis (see **Fig. 13**) due to spondylotic facet deformation. True spondilolisthesis due to isthmic lysis must be considered an absolute contraindication to use of such devices, because their action would widen and aggravate the lysis, not modify the degree of the olysthesis. Degenerative retrolisthesis with discopathy, reduction of the height of the posterior annulus, and possible associated Baastrup syndrome (kissing spinous processes with progressive, painful interspinous degenerative alteration) are good indications for an interspinous spacer.

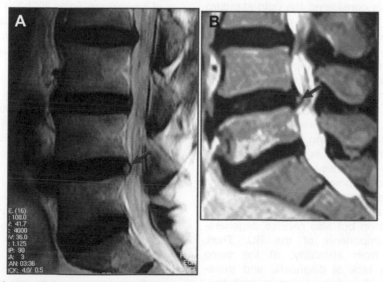

Fig. 16. (A and B) Hyperintensity zones in the posterior annulus, representing tears and granulation tissue (*arrows*). (B) Note the asymmetry of the outward bulging of the external, innervated fibers of the annulus, acting in compression rather than tension owing to nuclear degeneration (see text).

An osteoporotic condition must be considered a contraindication because of the risk of fractures consequent to the pressures generated against the bony surfaces.

SUMMARY

Dynamic stabilization (nonfusion or motion preservation technologies) aims to provide stabilization while maintaining the mobility and function of the SUs, favoring realignment; preventing extremes of flexion and extension; and unloading, through modification of distribution of loads, painful areas within the SU, especially disc or facets.

Dynamic unloading of the overall SU is not possible (it is equivalent to a rigid fusion). Often pain, however, is not from an increase of quantity of motion but from abnormal distribution of loads across sensitive areas of the SU. Changes in the location of the ICR change the deformation of local areas of tissue, moving the distribution of loading away from painful areas. Dynamic stabilization has the potential to relieve stress peaks in facets and anterior and posterior annulus, provided adequate spacer design and size are chosen. Thus, dynamic stabilization may provide pain relief by altering the transmission of abnormal loads across the degenerated structures.

Indications remain poorly defined, however, and largely reflect individual surgeon bias. The main issue is that current diagnostic techniques are not sufficient to identify the exact source of pain, and understanding of pain etiology is poor. The same issue underlies fusion surgery, however, which is considered the gold standard for treatment of instability. The dynamic stabilization techniques discussed in this article limit their therapeutic possibilities to lower grades of instability, thus representing a first, low-invasiveness tool in the armamentarium of the spine surgeon. Dynamic, minimally invasive implants should be used to avoid or delay more aggressive procedures, and their use as intermediate solutions is justified as long as the iatrogenic trauma during implantation is small. Low grades of instability are early ones and from a speculative and prospective point of view it is possible that an early correction of the problem, by means of minimally invasive, dynamic devices, could not only stop but also reverse degeneration of the components of the SU. Thus, patients suffer from instability; at the same time, there is a lack of diagnostic and therapeutic certainty. Far from being a limitation, this is the main advantage of dynamic stabilization systems, because they are minimally invasive, customizable, and easily reversible; maintain motion and spinal alignment; and are cheaper and safer than instrumented fusion procedures. And they do not burn down any bridges for further therapeutic options.

Most problems are still open and many questions are not yet answered. Further studies are required to determine optimal implants design. This is the beginning of a new era of surgery for the degenerated spine, requiring open minds and absence of biases. Radiologists are the best trained and culturally equipped for correct use and application of percutaneous or minimally invasive, often x-ray guided surgical techniques and devices. Many of these have been proposed and developed by radiologists. At the same time orthopedists and neurosurgeons share a long tradition of invasive treatments of the degenerated spine. The 2 worlds are getting closer, and an open and unbiased cooperation of the different communities should represent good news for our patients.

REFERENCES

1. Paris SV. Physical signs of instability. Spine 1985;10: 277–9.
2. Pope MH, Panjabi MM. Biomechanical definition of spine instability. Spine 1985;10:255–6.
3. American Academy of Orthopaedic Surgeons. A glossary on spinal terminology. Chicago: American Academy of Orthopaedic Surgeons; 1981.
4. Park P, Garton HJ, Gala VC, et al. Adjacent segment disease after lumbar or lumbosacral fusion: review of the literature. Spine 2004;29(17):1938–44.
5. Schlegel JD, Smith JA, Schleusener RL. Lumbar motion segment pathology adjacent to thoracolumbar, lumbar and lumbosacral fusions. Spine 1996; 21:970–81.
6. Aota Y, Kumano K, Hirabayashi S. Postfusion instability at the adjacent segments after rigid pedicle screw fixation for degenerative lumbar spinal disorders. J Spinal Disord 1995;8:464–73.
7. Etebar S, Cahill DW. Risk factors for adjacent-segment failure following lumbar fixation with rigid instrumentation for degenerative instability. J Neurosurg 1999;90:163–9.
8. Kumar MN, Jacquot F, Hall H. Long-term follow-up of functional outcomes and radiographic changes at adjacent levels following lumbar spine fusion for degenerative disc disease. Eur Spine J 2001;10: 309–13.
9. Hilibrand AS, Carlson GD, Palumbo MA, et al. Radiculopathy and myelopathy at segments adjacent to the site of a previous anterior cervical arthrodesis. J Bone Joint Surg Am 1999;81(4):519–28.

10. Ghiselli G, Wang JC, Bhatia NN, et al. Adjacent segment degeneration in the lumbar spine. J Bone Joint Surg Am 2004;86(7):1497–503.

11. Sengupta DK. Dynamic stabilization devices in the treatment of low back pain. Orthop Clin North Am 2004;35:43–56.

12. McNally DS. Rationale for dynamic stabilization. In: Kim D, Cammisa FP, Fessler RG, editors. Dynamic reconstruction of the spine. New York: Thieme; 2006. p. 237–43.

13. Wiseman C, Lindsey DP, Fredrick AD, et al. The effect of an interspinous process implant on facet loading during extension. Spine 2005;30:903–7.

14. Zucherman JF, Hsu KY, Hartjen CA, et al. A prospective randomized multi-center study for the treatment of lumbar spinal stenosis with the X-Stop interspinous implant: 1-year results. Eur Spine J 2004;13:22–31.

15. Katz JN, Harris MB. Lumbar spinal stenosis. N Engl J Med 2008;358:818–25.

16. Arbit E, Pannullo S. Lumbar stenosis: a clinical review. Clin Orthop 2001;384:137–43.

17. Blau JN, Logue V. The natural history of intermittent claudication of the cauda equina. A long term follow-up study. Brain 1978;101:211–22.

18. Lindsey DP, Swanson KE, Fuchs P, et al. The effects of an interspinous implant on the kinematics of the instrumented and adjacent levels in the lumbar spine. Spine 2003;28:2192–7.

19. Swanson KE, Lindsey DP, Hsu KY, et al. The effects of an interspinous implant on intervertebral disc pressures. Spine 2003;28:26–32.

20. Richards JC, Majumdar S, Lindsey DP, et al. The treatment mechanism of an interspinous process implant for lumbar neurogenic intermittent claudication. Spine 2005;30:744–9.

21. Zucherman JF, Hsu KY, Hartjen CA, et al. A multi-center, prospective, randomized trial evaluating the X STOP interspinous process decompression system for the treatment of neurogenic intermittent claudication. Two-year follow-up results. Spine 2005;30(12):1351–8.

22. Kondrashov DG, Hannibal M, Hsu KY, et al. Interspinous process decompression with the X-STOP device for lumbar spinal stenosis. A 4-Year follow-up study. J Spinal Disord Tech 2006;19(5):323–7.

23. Sénégas J, Etchevers JP, Baulny D, et al. Widening of the lumbar vertebral canal as an alternative to laminectomy, in the treatment of lumbar stenosis. Fr J Orthop Surg 1988;2:93–9.

24. Sénégas J. La ligamentoplastie intervertébrale, alternative à l'arthrodèse dans le traitement des instabilités dégénératives [Surgery of the intervertebral ligaments, alternative to arthrodesis in the treatment of degenerative instabilities]. Acta Orthop Belg 1991;57(Suppl 1):221–6 [in French].

25. Sénégas J. Mechanical supplementation by non-rigid fixation in degenerative intervertebral lumbar segments: the Wallis system. Eur Spine J 2002;11(Suppl 2):164–9.

26. Taylor J. Nonfusion technologies of the posterior column: a new posterior shock absorber. Presented at International Symposium on Intervertebral Disc Replacement and Non-Fusion-Technology. Munich, Germany, May 3 5, 2001.

27. Taylor J, Ritland S. Technical and anatomical considerations for the placement of a posterior interspinous stabilizer. In: Mayer HM, editor. Minimally invasive spine surgery. Berlin: Springer; 2006. p. 466–75.

28. Palmer S, Mahar A, Oka R. Biomechanical and radiographic analysis of a novel, minimally invasive, extension-limiting device for the lumbar spine. Neurosurg Focus 2007;22(1):1–6.

29. Siddiqui M, Nicol M, Karadimas E, et al. The positional magnetic resonance imaging changes in the lumbar spine following insertion of a novel interspinous process distraction device. Spine 2005;30:2677–82.

30. Siddiqui M, Karadimas E, Nicol M. Influence of X stop on neural foramina and spinal canal area in spinal stenosis. Spine 2006;31(25):2958–62.

31. Modic MT, Steinberg PM, Ross JS, et al. Degenerative disk disease: assessment of changes in vertebral body marrow with MR imaging. Radiology 1988;166(1pt1):193–9.

32. Aprill C, Bogduk N. High intensity zone: a diagnostic sign of painful lumbar disc on magnetic resonance imaging. Br J Radiol 1992;65:361–9.

33. Pfirrmann CW, Metzdorf A, Zanetti M, et al. Magnetic resonance classification of lumbar intervertebral disc degeneration. Spine 2001;26(17):1873–8.

Spinal Cord Stimulation: Uses and Applications

Stanley Golovac, MD

KEYWORDS

- Spinal cord • Neurostimulation • Spine anatomy
- Implantable spine stimulators
- Failed back spinal syndrome • Spine pain

Therapeutic electrical stimulation of the nervous system has developed enormously during the last 40 or so years, from the work that was performed by Shealy and colleagues[1] to the point where tens of thousands of units have been implanted every year, and yet one of the biggest criticisms is that there is a lack of high-quality evidence of its efficacy.

Since the recent enlightenment regarding the neurophysiology of pain, it has been discovered that electrical stimulation of almost any part of the nervous system can have a dramatic useful purpose of modulating painful conditions, such as spinal conditions (failed back spinal syndrome [FBSS]), complex regional pain syndrome (CRPS) I and II, interstitial cystitis, gastroparesis, chronic pancreatitis, peripheral neuropathic pain, and transformed migraine headaches. It seems that therapeutic stimulation has the potential to continue to add to the knowledge of neurologic function; for example, what does relief of central pain afforded by motor cortex stimulation tell about the integration of motor and sensory systems in the brain? It seems that, at least to some extent, spinal cord stimulation (SCS) influences the intrinsic, already available, modulatory systems, whose function may or may not have been disturbed, to bring about normalization. This principle may apply to neuropathic pain and maladaptive changes occurring in ischemic syndromes, such as myocardial ischemia, peripheral vascular ischemia, and neuropathic ischemia.

THE HISTORY OF NEUROSTIMULATION

Electrical stimulation for the treatment of pain has been around, in one form or another, in every culture for thousands of years. It is said that, from circa 9000 BC, bracelets were used to prevent headaches and arthritis.[2] Each culture acquired and/or discovered a type of fish that could, through electrical stimulation, stun or affect a person in one way or another. In the Nile Valley, Africa, electric catfish use electrical discharge to stun their prey. The ancient Egyptians acknowledged the power of the Nile catfish in tomb paintings. The ancient Greeks called the ray "Narke" or "numbness-producing," from which the word "narcosis" was coined. The Romans called the ray "torpedo" from the word "torpor" because the name was synonymous with the effect. Conditions such as gout and headaches were treated by having the torpedo fish discharge its electrical charge close to the site of the painful condition (**Fig. 1**).

The therapeutic application of electricity called "Franklinism" was named after the American statesman and scientist Benjamin Franklin, who, with his famous kite experiment in 1775, proved that lightening and electrostatic charge on a Leyden jar were identical. John Wesley, the founder of Methodism, extolled the virtues of electricity in his book, *The Desideratum*, and advocated electrotherapy for angina pectoris, gout, headaches, pleuritic pain, and sciatica.[3]

Disclosures: Consultant for Stryker Corporation & St. Jude Medical Neuro Division.
Space Coast Pain Institute, 595 North Courtenay Parkway, Merritt Island, FL 32953, USA
E-mail address: sgolovac@mac.com

Neuroimag Clin N Am 20 (2010) 243–254
doi:10.1016/j.nic.2010.02.012

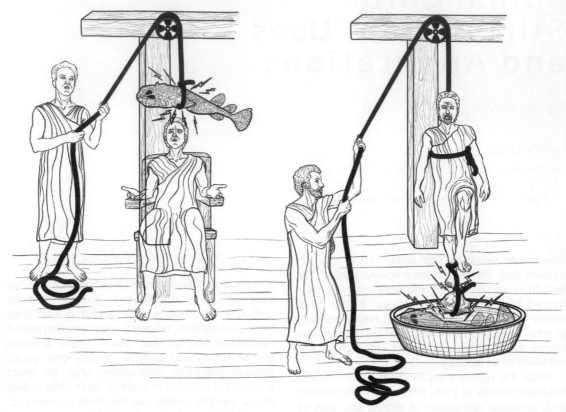

Fig. 1. Artist's impression of the treatment of gout (*left*) and headache (*right*) using torpedo fish. (*Adapted from* Perdikis P. Transcutaneous nerve stimulation in the treatment of protracted ileus. South African J Surg 1977;17(2):81–6; with permission.)

GATE CONTROL THEORY AND IMPLANTABLE STIMULATORS

The theory by Melzack and Wall[4] in 1965 postulated central inhibition of pain by nonpainful stimuli, a concept that had been predicted half a century ago by the English neurologist Sir Henry Head. In 1965, Wall recruited William Sweet, Head of Neurosurgery at Harvard Medical School, to clinically test the gate theory. Melzack and Wall proposed in their theory that nerve impulses from afferent fibers lead to spinal cord transmission (T) cells in the substantia gelatinosa. The firing of the projection neuron determines pain. The inhibitory interneuron decreases the chance that the projection neuron will fire. Firing of C fibers inhibits the inhibitory interneuron (indirectly), thereby increasing the chances that the projection neuron will fire. Firing of the large myelinated Aβ fibers activates the inhibitory interneuron, reducing the chances that the projection neuron will fire, even in the presence of a firing nociceptive fiber. The marriage of electricity to pain control in this paradigm of the gate control theory lies in the age-old

principle of "counterirritation." At first, they experimented on their own infraorbital nerves using needle-stimulating electrodes and on superficial nerves, such as the ulnar nerve, using superficial electrodes. Then they used transcutaneous or percutaneous stimulation in 3 patients who experienced partial or complete relief of pain during stimulation.[4,5] Shealy (a neurosurgeon in La Crosse, Wisconsin) and colleagues[6] thought that the "gate" could be best closed by stimulating the dorsal columns and confirmed this assumption experimentally in cats. In 1967, Shealy and his coworkers implanted a device (**Fig. 2**) in a 50-year-old woman suffering from intractable carcinomatous pelvic pain and used a radiofrequency stimulator.[6]

The circuit design was based on a modified Medtronic device (Medtronic, Inc, Minneapolis, MN, USA) for the stimulation of the carotid sinus to control angina and hypertension. The patient experienced approximately 50% relief from her pain, at times almost total control of her pain, and was extensively evaluated until Mortimer

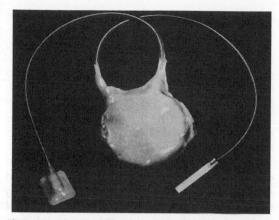

Fig. 2. Bottom view of assembled radiofrequency receiver and electrodes as implanted in Shealy's second patient on October 8, 1967. The coiled platinum-iridium wires connecting the electrodes to the receiver and the epoxy and glass portions of the receiver were covered with medical grade Silastic. The system was activated by a variable frequency transmitter-stimulator with a fixed pulse width. Frequency and amplitude were controlled by the patient. (*Reprinted from* Mortimer JT. Pain suppression in man by dorsal column electroanalgesia [PhD thesis]. Case Western Reserve University, Cleveland, OH, USA; with permission.)

(from Shealy's team) successfully defended his PhD thesis *Pain suppression in man by dorsal column electroanalgesia* in May 1968.[1]

DORSAL ROOTS

Most dorsal root fibers, on entering the spinal cord, proceed toward the dorsal columns, where they bifurcate into ascending and descending branches.[7,8] In comparison with longitudinal dorsal column fibers, dorsal root fibers have a curved shape, and they differ in orientation with respect to the spinal cord and the implanted electrodes. Dorsal root fibers average 15 μm in diameter. Proximal to the dorsal ganglion, the dorsal root fibers fan-out in an ascending, dorsomedial direction to form the rootlets that enter the spinal cord at different angles. Strujik and colleagues[9] have studied the effect of the curvature of the dorsal roots on their electrical threshold.[10,11]

CHRONIC BACK PAIN

Back pain is responsible for more than 80% of all back pain syndromes affecting Americans daily. One in every 14 individuals is affected by some kind of cervical, thoracic, or lumbar pain, meaning that out-of-work days can affect the work status of employers. Estimated annual cost for direct and indirect treatments is 20 to 60 billion dollars annually.[12]

Most types of back pain are acute or subacute, resolving within a 6-week period of time normally. However, other estimates suggest that less than 30% of patients are completely improved within 3 months of treatment.[13]

Chronic low back pain represents one of the most widespread and costly medical problems today; it is also a major cause of workplace absenteeism. Past analyses have demonstrated that more than 5 million people in the United States are afflicted with chronic low back pain. Conservative estimates place the annual cost of treatment at 25 billion dollars.[14] A significant fraction of these dollars is attributable to more than 200,000 US patients yearly who elect for lumbosacral surgery to relieve their pain. Unfortunately, 20% to 40% of surgical patients experience persistent or recurrent pain.[15]

Failed Back Spinal Syndrome

One important subset of patients includes those with the so-called failed back surgery syndrome. In the literature, this multidimensional syndrome has been used to describe various types of pain, including centrally located lumbosacral pain, buttock pain, gluteal pain, extremity pain, and diffuse lower back pain. Many published series emphasize the distinction between back pain and leg pain; however, details of the pain syndromes are usually lacking. The cause of these pains is very difficult to pinpoint. Some of the reasons are wrong level of surgery, psychological overlay, arachnoiditis, lumbosacral epidural fibrosis, vertebral microinstability, and recurrent disk herniations.

Although there are several paths as to why one develops a condition such as FBSS, the most common, unfortunately, is the poor selection for the surgery. This means that the patient may have had a psychological profile or physical pathology that was contraindicated or not appropriate for the surgical intervention.[16,17] Furthermore, if the patient is misdiagnosed, the surgery is obviously incorrect and damaging. The most common misdiagnosis in these cases is arthritis misdiagnosed as lumbar disk disease. Often, improper selection and misdiagnosis follow from inadequate preoperative evaluation and diagnosis workup. A full diagnostic workup should include a medical and psychological evaluation. The medical evaluation should include a comprehensive physical examination and history, imaging, and relevant diagnostic procedures, such as radiography, computed tomography, magnetic resonance imaging, myelography, bone scanning, electromyography, discography, and various diagnostic injections, to help delineate the pain generator.[18]

Surgery that is unnecessary may also be the cause of FBSS. Unnecessary surgery not only fails to treat the problem appropriately but also may worsen the patient's condition. An unnecessary surgical excision of the nucleus pulposus from the normal disk is likely to increase the risk of chronic back pain by creating instability and malalignment. Needless surgery places patients at unnecessary risk for injured nerves, torn dura or arachnoid, cerebrospinal fluid (CSF) leakage, and later for possible wound infection or hemorrhage.[19]

Complex Regional Pain Syndrome

CRPS, formerly recognized as reflex sympathetic dystrophy, is frequently misunderstood, misdiagnosed, and mistreated. First and foremost, reestablishing the function of the injured area is of utmost importance. Only 1 in 5 is able to return to work after having been diagnosed with the disease. It has been estimated to occur in approximately 1:2000 traumatic events.[20] In 1994, the International Association for the Study of Pain proposed stringent diagnostic criteria and named the "complex regional pain syndrome type I."[21] Pain alleviation is secondary when it comes to the function of the injured area. As one of the author's colleagues says frequently, "this is not a disease of the extremity; it is a disease of the nervous system."

Initial work performed by the late Bonica[22] provides an explanation of the disease-development stages. Stage 1, or the acute phase, is when the extremity is very sensitive to any form of touch, contact, or stimulus. The extremity may seem swollen, discolored, and stiff. Stage 2, or the dystrophic phase, is seen some 3 to 4 months after the initial injury. During this stage, the extremity begins to become contracted and remains swollen and very painful. The area now begins to feel cooler with respect to the other extremity. Unfortunately, during Stage 3, or the atrophic phase, the extremity becomes almost useless. If severe atrophy develops, uncal changes occur. Brittle nails form, and either excessive hair growth or sparse hair can result.

Physical therapy is mandatory to even hope for any improvement of the injured area. Functionality is the key. The injured area should respond to a combination of treatments. Medications should be started to improve sleep and inhibit neuropathic impulses from the injury; sympathetic inhibition is important to restore blood flow to the injury.

Conventional pain medication, physical therapy, sympathetic blocks, and transcutaneous electrostimulation of the nerves have all been used to help alleviate pain caused by the initial injury. SCS introduced by Shealy and colleagues[6] in 1967 has been one of the most successful modalities used for alleviating pain, swelling, and stiffness today.

Of extreme importance in the clinical application of SCS to complex pain syndromes was that multiple arrays of electrodes with defined spacing would allow "capture" of pain (ie, the overlap of areas of paresthesia over the region of pain perception) better than a single array of electrodes.[1,20,21,23–29] Law and Kirkpatrick[30] showed that a defined area of the spinal cord, the physiologic midline, which differed from the anatomic midline, was crucial in the modulation of pain transmission. They also determined that medial dorsal column penetration was improved with bilaterally placed electrode arrays around the physiologic midline using staggered guarded cathodes with intercontact spacing of 4 mm and surface contact of 3 mm. (A guarded cathode is a selection of 3 adjacent electrodes with the midline electrode, the cathode [negative], having opposite polarity from the surrounding 2 anodal [positive] electrodes.) This would enhance the capture of pain in complex dynamic pain syndrome with axial back pain and CRPS. The concept of dual arrays of electrodes led the way to multichannel devices that allow the steering of paresthesia (ie, the moving of the active cathode in the longitudinal and transverse directions electronically) without the need for surgical intervention. A multichannel device (Fig. 3) is one that allows for more than one lead to be active simultaneously, thus increasing the area of the spinal cord that can be covered.

As soon as the pain improves, swelling, trophic changes, and function should begin to improve. The pseudomotor changes that were initially seen then begin to return to preinjury states. Care should always be stressed with relation to the use of the extremity, but one should never treat the injured extremity differently with respect to its daily use. One should force the extremity to function normally.

ARACHNOIDITIS

Arachnoiditis is a postsurgical complication and is believed to be caused by scarring and adhesions located intraspinally. Because of the phenomenon that develops, pain from the adhesions and

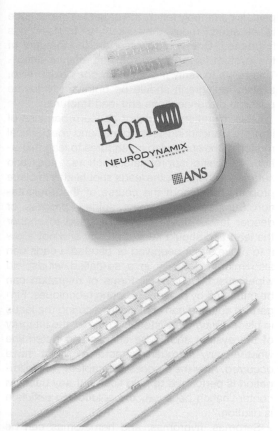

Fig. 3. Multichannel device. (*Courtesy of* St. Jude Medical, St. Paul, MN; with permission; image copyright St. Jude Medical, all rights reserved.)

clumping cause pain with movement of the spine, dysesthetic burning pain in extremities, and loss of functionality. Once again, this unfortunate painful syndrome has very few solutions to its treatment. Intrathecal pain-alleviating medications can be used, but, as has been frequently witnessed, this modality leads only to dependency, tolerance, and habituation.

OCCIPITAL NEURALGIA (PERIPHERAL NERVE STIMULATOR)

Occipital neuralgia is characterized by paroxysms of pain occurring within the distribution of the greater occipital nerves. The pain may radiate to the ipsilateral frontal or retro-orbital regions of the head. Extreme localized tenderness is often encountered upon palpation over the occipital notches, with reproduction of focal and radiating pain. Though known causes include closed head trauma, direct occipital nerve injury, neuroma formation, or upper cervical nerve root compression (spondylosis or ligamentous hypertrophy), most patients have no demonstrable lesions.

Treatment options for intractable occipital nerve pain refractory to medications usually involve chemical, thermal, or surgical ablation, after diagnostic local anesthetic blockade. Surgical approaches include neurolysis or nerve sectioning.[1]

ANGINA PECTORIS AND PERIPHERAL VASCULAR DISEASE

In 1999, the American Heart Association defined angina pectoris as a clinical syndrome characterized by discomfort in the chest, jaw, shoulder, back, or arm, typically aggravated by stress.[31–34] The syndrome is caused by an imbalance between demand and supply of oxygen to the heart. The decrease in blood supply to the heart is usually the result of vessel occlusion or vasospasm. An angina attack is triggered by an increased demand for oxygen caused by physical stresses. Heart disease remains the leading cause of death in the United States and contributes extensively to health care costs to society.

The most common group of patients with refractory angina pectoris has coronary artery disease that is not corrected by bypass grafting, stent placement, or aggressive medical management. Another group of refractory patients demonstrates normal coronary angiographies but has significant intermittent angina discomfort.

This condition is sometimes referred to as microvascular disease or small vessel disease. On exercise electrocardiogram, the patients have typical exercise-triggered angina with ST segment depression. Because they generally fail to respond to conventional antiangina therapy, they remain a treatment dilemma. Some of the theories as to the cause of this syndrome include endothelial dysfunction, abnormal distribution and function of adenosine receptors, and estrogen deficiency. These are the treatment dilemmas for the cardiac team.

Ischemic changes occur as a result of the sympathetic inhibition that allows for more blood to flow in the ischemic areas. This then allows for the peripheral circulation to improve cellular activity and overall blood flow. By inhibiting circulating catecholamine, the circulatory system behaves by producing a vasodilatory effect, thereby allowing more nutrients to flow to areas that are deprived of vital nutrients that allow cellular activity to function without forming lactic acidosis and increasing pain in the ischemic area.

TECHNICAL FACTORS IN SCS

Spinal cord stimulation is a procedure that must be performed under fluoroscopic guidance.

Understanding the three dimensional views of the spinal canal and the anatomy is crucial to proper insertion and alleviation of pain at the site of the target. Proper sterile technique needs to be adhered to. Gown and gloves should be used, and sterile preparation with Betadine and alcohol should take place to create a sterile field for insertion. Proper antibiotic should be administered and proper time allowed for adequate circulating levels to ensure tissue-level coverage from the antibiotic administered. Mask and sterile technique are essential to prevent infections from developing. The patient is placed on a well-padded carbon fiber fluoroscopic table to allow full-field visualization of the spine in an anterior-posterior and a lateral view.

Understanding of anatomic placement allows the implanter to access the epidural space with ease. This allows for insertion of 1, 2, 3, or 4 leads with less difficulty.

With placing, 1, 2, 3, and even 4 leads can be inserted into the epidural space, either from an anterograde or from a retrograde manner. This allows stimulation over the sacral plexus. By stimulating the sacral 2, 3, and 4 nerve rootlets, one can inhibit afferent impulses from entering the dorsal cord painfully.

COMPLICATIONS

Complications include wound infections, lead fractures, inadvertent spinal taps, epidural punctures, lead migrations, inability to cover the area desired, seromas, hygromas, hematomas, and spinal cord trauma. An infection can develop each and every time the skin barrier is violated. The most common infections seen and dealt with are those caused by *Staphylococcus aureus*. *Staphylococcus epidermidis* is another well-known felon. In this era of resistant bacteria, coverage for resistant strains of bacteria needs to be considered in addition to simple everyday bacterial coverage. Methicillin-resistant *S aureus* is becoming a common bacterium, one that is difficult to eradicate because of the super infections that have developed from overuse/misuse of antibiotics. Sterile precautions need to be taken each and every time the skin barrier is violated. Proper prepping and draping is essential for the prevention of microbacteria contamination. Gowning and gloving and adherence to a sterile technique are imperative. Even with these measures, widespread infections are occurring.

Lead fractures and interruption in conductivity are issues that need to be looked into when coverage is interrupted. Pain at the site of the fracture is typically seen. Dysesthesia, a burning-type pain, is commonly felt by the patient. If impedance is elevated, more than likely a fracture has happened. One way to ascertain the integrity of the system is to perform an impedance check. This helps to verify if a problem does exist. Also, a plain radiograph should be obtained to locate possible disconnections and lead fractures.

Lead migration is a major concern because of improper anchoring techniques, and mechanical motion of the spine also contributes to lead migration. By using appropriate anchors, glue, and suturing techniques, the leads should stay in place properly throughout the course of the implantation. Supraspinous ligament, spinous process, or deeper fascial tissue should be used to anchor the lead and should keep it steady and not allow it to move either cephalad or caudad. Leads can also migrate laterally in a so-called windshield wiper effect. Usually, all forms of migration can be mitigated by proper anchoring techniques. Fingertrap suturing can also aid in securing the leads in place. Once the system is in place, the integrity of the system should be checked to determine whether any iatrogenic fractures might have occurred. After the process is complete, ample irrigation is performed to help flush out any bacteria contamination because "the solution to pollution is dilution."

Seromas, hygromas, and hematomas can be avoided by strict hemostasis techniques and also by creating a pocket that is adequate for the battery device that is being implanted. Not allowing excessive motion and contact between the interface of the battery and the subcutaneous tissue minimizes any chance of seroma formation.

Along with the previously mentioned complications, there are several other complications that can develop, including a dural tear, CSF leak, cord compression from either a trauma from the lead insertion or an unrecognized spinal canal stenosis that develops from iatrogenic causes, infection, inability to obtain the desired results, lead movement or migration, persistent pain from dural irritation, seromas, hygromas, rejection and allergic reactions, local skin erosions, paralysis or weakness, and pain at implant site.

TECHNIQUES AND PEARLS OF IMPLANTATION

Patient positioning is a major key element in accurately inserting a lead into the epidural space. A large pillow should be placed under the pelvic brim for men and under the abdomen for women. By reversing the lumbar lordosis, the interlaminar spaces open to their widest space. This allows easier access into the epidural space for the insertion needle. A 30° angle into the epidural space is desired. The typical way to enter is by starting 1 interlaminar space below the targeted entrance site. Then, after anesthetizing a tract down to the lamina, use an 18-gauge needle or a No. 11 blade to nick the skin. After this, use the bubble technique and the loss of resistance technique with a pulsator syringe with saline. Enter the epidural space, and use some saline to expand the space. Then guide the lead up to the desired level of dermatomal coverage. Steering can be performed in various ways and each implanter develops techniques that allow the procedure to be performed smoothly. After proper anterior and lateral views to determine posterior epidural lead placement, connect the leads to the testing cables and begin the stimulation process to evaluate the adequate paresthesia coverage over the painful zone and desired relief (Fig. 4).

If a lead meets resistance and cannot be advanced, then a simple technique of retracting the inner guidewire approximately 2 to 3 cm from the tip can be performed. Twirl the lead while advancing the lead forward. This may be sufficient to redirect the lead in the direction desired. Lead location is determined by the segment of the spinal cord that correlates to the anatomic area of dorsal column fibers located throughout the spinal cord.

Anchoring is another crucial and important part of the procedure. There are several types of anchors that can be used. Different products advocate the use of specific types of anchors, from the hard anchor to the bumpy and the sleeve types. Each allows for a suture to be placed around the lead. Then it is secured to the fascia between the ligaments. Some products even advocate the use of a glue to help secure the lead to the anchor. There is even a technique of simply securing the lead to the subcutaneous tissue without an anchor to hold the lead. This allows for some movement to occur when the patient either flexes or extends.

Tunneling and generator placement are the next steps. Proper depth and location need to be considered in order not to encounter an irritative source such as a belt or an object when the patient sits. Proper depth is crucial with rechargeable units. If the battery is too deep, then contact will not occur, and the battery will not be able to engage for recharging. If the battery is placed too superficial, then the contact area may produce dysesthetic phenomena at the site of contact (Fig. 5).

Landmarks are crucial for precise placement. First, identify the anatomic midline. Aligning the spinous process, pedicles, and endplates of the entrance site allows for an easier placement. The lamina should be as open as possible. Remember that reversing the lordosis in the lumbar area allows for this to occur. The 12th rib is also a point of reference.

The anatomic midline and the physiologic midline are 2 different areas. One may not coincide

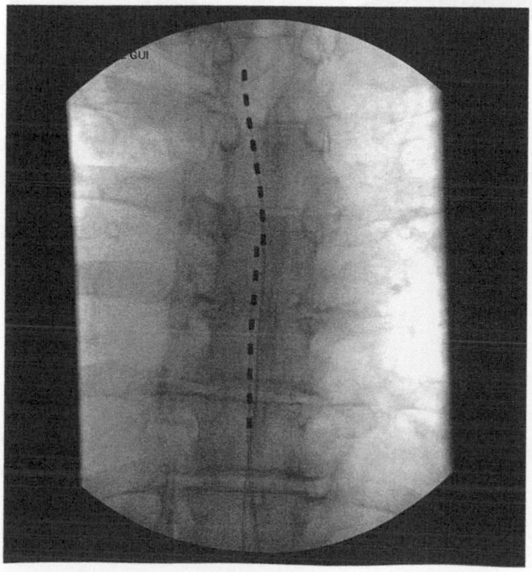

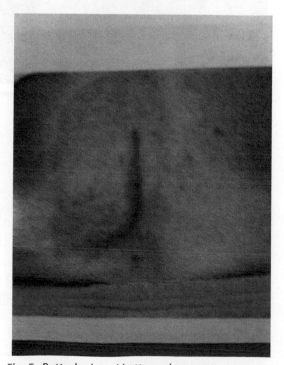

Fig. 4. Stimulation lead configuration.

Fig. 5. Buttock gluteal battery placement.

with the other. One should gauge oneself via the anatomic one first, but be ready to steer the leads off the midline if the patient does not perceive stimulation. The spinal cord can twist and turn throughout its course and not correlate to the anatomic midline.

After all is said and done, confirm impedance before closing the wound to save the painstaking time required to revise a freshly placed stimulator.

Lead placement and configuration depends on a patient's pain pattern (**Fig. 6**). Each patient designs his/her own lead configuration by indicating to the implanter where his/her pain is perceived and how the distribution of the pain pattern can be covered. Midline cervical pain patterns can be covered with a single lead array.

Dual cervical lead placement can also be used for several reasons: for lead stabilization, for using a guarded cathode configuration, and for allowing a broader coverage area with 2 leads. Mid to upper thoracic lead placement can be used for angina, midepigastric pain and pancreatic pain. Lumbar lead placement is typically located between the T8 and T10 area midline in the thoracic spine.

DEVICE MANUFACTURERS

Three companies offer devices for implantation: Medtronic, Inc (Minneapolis, MN, USA) (the oldest), St. Jude Medical (St. Paul, MN, USA), and Boston Scientific (Natick, MA, USA). All these

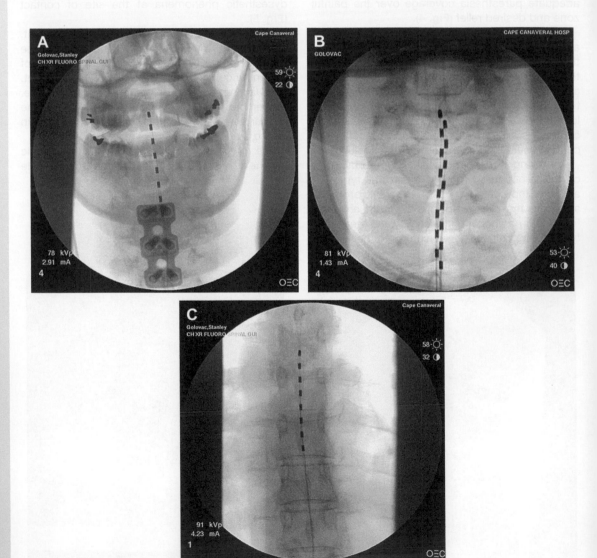

Fig. 6. (A–C) Lead placement.

A

B

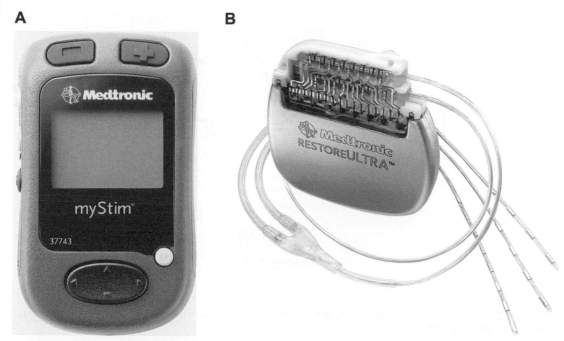

Fig. 7. Medtronic's patient programmer (*A*) used with its RestoreUltra neurostimulation system (*B*). (*Courtesy of* Medtronic, Inc, Minneapolis, MN; with permission.)

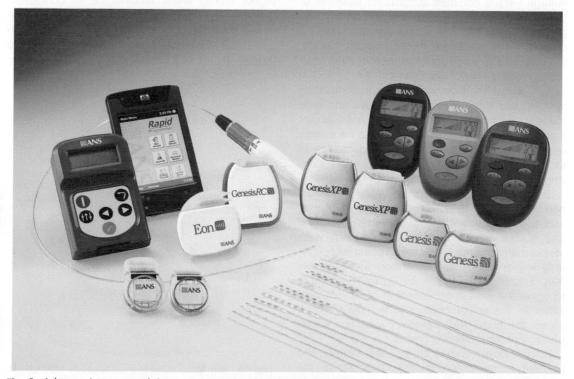

Fig. 8. Advanced Neuromodulation Systems product family. (*Courtesy of* St. Jude Medical, St. Paul, MN; with permission; image copyright St. Jude Medical, all rights reserved.)

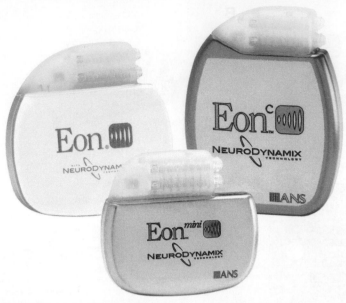

Fig. 9. Eon, Eon Mini, EonC. (*Courtesy of* St. Jude Medical, St. Paul, MN; with permission; image copyright St. Jude Medical, all rights reserved.)

companies have very good products, but each has 1 item that the other does not have.

Medtronic uses a voltage called constant voltage versus constant current. An example of this is when a car is placed on cruise control and ascends up a hill, the accelerator increases to overcome the resistance. As for constant voltage, the voltage stays constant, the current does not.

Medtronic's handheld programmer (**Fig.** 7A) (used with its RestoreUltra neurostimulation system, see **Fig.** 7B) is simple to use and user friendly. Having a set of controls in hand allows a patient to easily increase or decrease the energy requirements that he or she may need, as well as to move the stimulation up and down the electrodes to maximize pain control.

St. Jude Medical offers an array of leads, paddles, steering devices, rechargeable batteries, and constant current energy deliverance (**Figs.** 8 and 9). The newest addition to an already well-stocked armamentarium is the smallest rechargeable implantable pulse generator, the Eon Mini (**Fig.** 10), which can allow for up to 16 contacts to cover the area in question that generates pain either in the spinal cord or in the periphery. It allows for longer rechargeable cycles and easier placement for patients' comfort.

Boston Scientific has the smallest battery and i-Sculpt technology (**Fig.** 11). This allows the programmer to shift the energy from one lead to another and cover certain areas.

Energy is the limiting factor, meaning the more the device is used, the less the battery life it will have. With the rechargeable system, one can use higher energy levels and not be as concerned with the battery life. All battery lives do end at some point. Medtronic's battery ends at the 9-year mark. St. Jude Medical has been able to extend the life of its battery to 10 years or more,

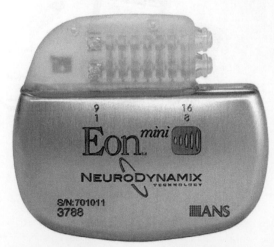

Fig. 10. Eon Mini. (*Courtesy of* St. Jude Medical, St. Paul, MN; with permission; image copyright St. Jude Medical, all rights reserved.)

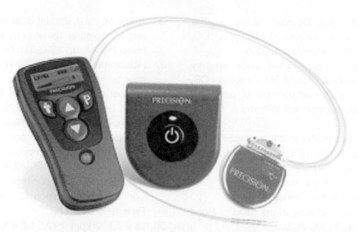

Fig. 11. Precision plus system. (*Courtesy of* Boston Scientific, Natick, MA; with permission.)

and Boston Scientific's battery ends at approximately the 5-year mark.

SUMMARY

SCS can provide significant long-term pain relief and improve quality of life in a variety of benign intractable pain-generating causes. The most beneficial effects are noted in the cases of FBSS, CRPS I and II, pain secondary to peripheral vascular disease, angina, multiple sclerosis, and peripheral neuropathy. In addition to improvements in pain intensity, patients also reported increases in social interactions, mood elevation, and various factors in daily living. SCS using multipolar and multichannel stimulation programs have improved long-term success rates significantly in comparison with the previous decade. The use of multiple leads allowing multiple electrode combinations and sophisticated programming seems to hold much promise in the treatment of patients with predominantly axial back pain, which in the past has been resistant to SCS therapy. The complication rate is low, which makes SCS a safe and effective approach in the management of long-term pain. The concept of tolerance continues to be the most significant challenge to long-term efficacy of SCS therapy, and further work is required to elucidate its pathophysiology. Prospective randomized controlled studies that are currently in progress will further confirm these conclusions.

REFERENCES

1. Shealy CM, Mortimer JT, Reswick JB. Electrical inhibition of pain by stimulation of the dorsal columns. Anesth Analg 1967;46:489–91.
2. Schechter DC. Origins of electrotherapy. I. N Y State J Med 1971;71(9):997–1008.
3. Gadsby JG. Electroanalgesia: historical and contemporary development [PhD thesis]. Leicester (UK): De Montfort University; 1998.
4. Melzack R, Wall PD. Pain mechanisms: a new theory. Science 1965;250:971–8.
5. Wall PD, Sweet WH. Temporary abolition of pain in man. Science 1967;155:108–9.
6. Shealy CN, Taclitz N, Mortimer JT, et al. Electrical inhibition of pain: experimental evaluation. Anesth Analg 1967;46(3):299–305.
7. Davidoff RA. Handbook of spinal cord, vols. 2 and 3. New York: Marcel Dekker Inc; 1984.
8. Carpenter MB. Human neuroanatomy. Baltimore (MD): Williams & Wilkins; 1976.
9. Strujik JJ, Holsheimer J, Boom HB. Excitation of dorsal root fibers in spinal cord stimulation: a theoretical study. IEEE Trans Biomed Eng 1993;40:632–8.
10. Strujik JJ, Holsheimer J, van Veen BK, et al. Epidural spinal cord stimulation: calculation of field potentials with special reference to dorsal column nerve fibers. IEEE Trans Biomed Eng 1991;38:104–10.
11. Strujik JJ, Holsheimer J. Transverse tripole spinal cord stimulation: theoretical performance of a dual channel system. Med Biol Eng Comput 1996;34:273–9.
12. Mayer TG, Gatchel RJ. Functional restoration for spinal disorders: the sports medicine approach Philadelphia. Philadelphia: Lea & Febiger; 1988.
13. Croft PR, Joseph S, Cosgrove S, et al. Low back pain in the community and hospitals. Report to the Clinical Standards Advisory Group of the Department of Health, 1994.
14. Frymoyer JW, Cats-Baril WL. An overview of the incidences and costs of low back pain. Orthop Clin North Am 1991;22:263–71.
15. Wilkinson HA. The failed back syndrome: etiology and therapy. 2nd edition. Philadelphia: Harper and Row; 1991.

16. Block AR, Gatchel RJ, Deardoff W, et al. The psychology of spine surgery. Washington, DC: American Psychology Association; 2003.

17. Oaklander AI, North RB. Failed back surgery syndrome. In: Loeser JD, Butler SH, Chapman CR, et al, editors. Bonica's management of pain. 3rd edition. Philadelphia: Lippincott Williams & Wilkins; 2001.

18. Green LN. Dexamethasone in the management of symptoms due to herniated lumbar disc. J Neurol Neurosurg Psychiatry 1975;38:1211–7.

19. Wilkinson HA. The failed back syndrome. 2nd edition. New York: Springer-Verlag; 1992.

20. Plewes LW. Sudecks atrophy in the hand. J Bone Joint Surg Br 1956;38:195–203.

21. Merskey H, Bogduk N. Classification of chronic pain: descriptions of chronic pain syndromes and definitions of pain terms. 2nd edition. Seattle (WA): IASP Press; 1994. p. 40–2.

22. Bonica J. Causalgia and other reflex sympathetic dystrophys. In: Bonica J, Liebeskinar J, Albe-Fessard D, editors. Advances in pain research and therapy: proceedings of the second world congress on pain. New York: Raven Press; 1979. p. 141–66.

23. Law JD. Spinal stimulation: statistical superiority of monophasic stimulation of narrowly separated, longitudinal bipoles having rostral cathodes. Appl Neurophysiol 1983;46:129–37.

24. Law JD. A new method for targeting a spinal stimulator: quantitatively paired comparisons. Appl Neurophysiol 1987;50:436.

25. Law JD. Clinical and technical results from spinal stimulation for chronic pain of diverse pathologies. Stereotact Funct Neurosurg 1992;59:21–4.

26. Tulgar M, He J, Barolat G, et al. Analysis of parameters for epidural spinal cord stimulation. Stereotact Funct Neurosurg 1993;61:146–55.

27. Holsheimer J, Strujik JJ, Rijkhoff NJ. Contact combinations in epidural spinal cord stimulation. A comparison by computer modeling. Stereotact Funct Neurosurg 1991;56:220–33.

28. Holsheimer J, Strujik JJ. How do geometric factors influence epidural spinal cord stimulation? Quantitative analyses by computer modeling. Stereotact Funct Neurosurg 1991;56:234–49.

29. He J, Barolat G, Holsheimer J. Perception threshold and electrode position for spinal cord simulation. Pain 1994;59:55–63.

30. Law JD, Kirkpatrick AF. Intractable pain of both arms and legs can be treated with complex spinal cord stimulation. Abstract of the 7th World Congress on Pain. Seattle (WA): IASP Publications; 1993. p. 422.

31. Gibbons RJ, Chatterjee K, Daley J, et al. ACC/AHA/ACP-ASIm guidelines for the management of patients with chronic stable angina: a report of the American College of Cardiology/Heat Association Task Force on Practice Guidelines. J Am Coll Cardiol 1999;33:2092–197.

32. Feler CA, Whitworth LA, Brookoff D, et al. Recent advances: sacral nerve root stimulation using a retrograde method of lead insertion for the treatment of pelvic pain due to interstitial cystitis. Neuromodulation 1999;2:211–6.

33. Jones CA, Nyberg LM. Epidemiology of interstitial cystitis. Urology 1997;49:2–9.

34. Koziol JA, Clark DC, Gittes RF, et al. The natural history of interstitial cystitis-a survey of 374 patients. J Urol 1993;149:465–9.

Index

Note: Page numbers of article titles are in **boldface** type.

Moving?

Make sure your subscription moves with you!

To notify us of your new address, find your **Clinics Account Number** (located on your mailing label above your name), and contact customer service at:

Email: journalscustomerservice-usa@elsevier.com

800-654-2452 (subscribers in the U.S. & Canada)
314-447-8871 (subscribers outside of the U.S. & Canada)

Fax number: 314-447-8029

Elsevier Health Sciences Division
Subscription Customer Service
3251 Riverport Lane
Maryland Heights, MO 63043

*To ensure uninterrupted delivery of your subscription, please notify us at least 4 weeks in advance of move.

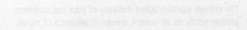

Printed and bound by CPI Group (UK) Ltd, Croydon, CR0 4YY

03/10/2024

01040359-0013